Reflections

Learning English through Real Nursing Stories

看護師たちの
リフレクション

医療現場のストーリーで学ぶ英語

Yoshifumi Tanaka

SANSHUSHA

音声ダウンロード＆ストリーミングサービス（無料）のご案内

https://www.sanshusha.co.jp/text/onsei/isbn/9784384335194/

本書の音声データは、上記アドレスよりダウンロードおよびストリーミング再生ができます。ぜひご利用ください。

Download

Streaming

はしがき

　米国の看護学専門誌 *American Journal of Nursing*（1900 年創刊）に *Reflections* という名称のコラム欄が誕生したのは 1983 年のことです。「リフレクション」（reflection）とは，一般的には「内省，省察」と訳されますが，看護の分野では「日々の看護実践に対する客観的な振り返り」を指します。同誌のこのコラム欄に掲載される短いエッセイは，大半が看護師によるものですが，そのほかの医療従事者，患者やその家族も執筆しています。誕生と同時に大人気を博したこのコラム欄に掲載されたエッセイは，*Reflections on Nursing: 80 Inspiring Stories on the Art and Science of Nursing*（2017）として刊行されました。本書は，この書籍に収録された 80 編から選りすぐった 15 編のエッセイをもとに作成した，主に看護学生向けの英語学習用テキストです。

　各 Unit の構成は次のようになっています。

WARM UP　　Vocabulary & Pronunciation

本文に出てくる単語の意味を確認して，発音を練習します。

READING

医療・看護分野の単語・重要表現については本文右側に注が付けてあります。一般的な単語・重要表現や構文については脚注が付けてあります。

Essay【Part 1】 エッセイの出だしを読み，**Check the situation** で場面を確認してください。
Essay【Part 2】 エッセイの続きを読み，**Reading Comprehension** で本文の内容を確認してください。

EXERCISES　　Dictation & Translation

音声を聴いて英文の空欄を補充し，完成した英文を日本語に直す問題です。注で取り上げた重要表現を確認してください。

EXERCISES　　Word Order & Translation

日本語を参考にして英文を作る問題です。注で取り上げた重要表現や構文を確認してください。音声を聴いて英文を確認することも可能です。

Nursing Terms and Expressions

看護の分野で重要な単語や表現を確認する問題です。

Column

医療や看護の分野の「ことばと文化」を取り上げています。

　収録されたエッセイが看護職者をめざすみなさんの心に響き，本書がみなさんの英語学習に少しでも役立つことを願っています。

2022 年秋
編著者

Contents

資格・略称一覧

以下はエッセイを記した米国の看護師たちの資格・略称です。

ASN	Associate of Science in Nursing
BSN	Bachelor of Science in Nursing
CNOR	Certified Nurse Operating Room
CNS-BC	Clinical Nurse Specialist-Board Certified
CPN	Certified Pediatric Nurse
CPNP	Certified Pediatric Nurse Practitioner
CRNP	Certified Registered Nurse Practitioner
FAAN	Fellow of the American Academy of Nursing
MA	Master of Arts
MD	Doctor of Medicine
MEd	Master of Education
MPH	Master of Public Health
MS	Master of Science
MSN	Master of Science in Nursing
PCCN	Progressive Care Certified Nurse
PhD	Doctor of Philosophy
PMH-NP	Psychiatric Mental Health-Nurse Practitioner
PNP-BC	Pediatric Nurse Practitioner-Board Certified
RN	Registered Nurse
RN-BC	Registered Nurse-Board Certified

Unit 1
No Regrets

There is such a thing as a good death.

Arlene Koch, RN

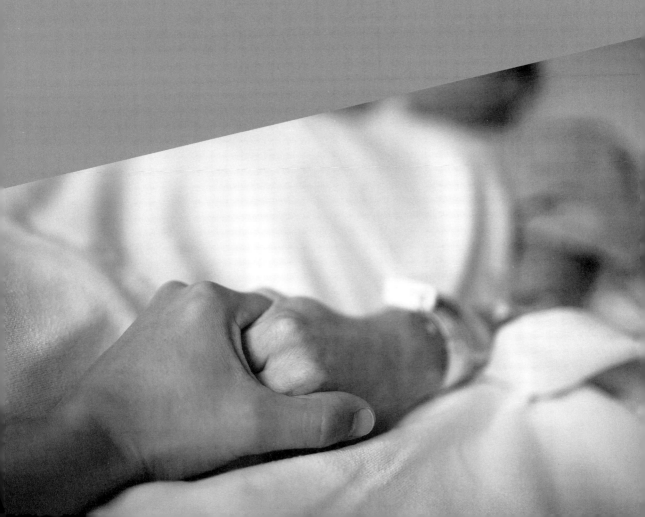

次の英語の意味に合う日本語を下から選びなさい。また，音声を聴いて発音しなさい。

1. bowel _____

2. abdomen _____

3. guarantee _____

4. anticipate _____

5. deteriorate _____

保証する，腹部，衰える，予想する，腸

READING   **Essay【Part 1】**   CD 1-02 ▶ 02

エッセイの出だしを読んでみましょう。

Medical and Nursing Notes

Ray Troyan was curled in the fetal position, rocking back and forth. A severely perforated bowel caused him so much pain that on a 1-to-10 scale, he rated it a 20. He was 87 years old and had been admitted 48 hours earlier with chest pain, but now the
5 pain was localized in his abdomen. His daughter, Kathryn, had been called in during the night. Neither of them had slept.

Ray had to make a choice. If he chose surgery, it would have to be done immediately. Not having surgery would mean death. Ray's age and the magnitude of the surgery were two
10 factors working against him. The surgeons couldn't guarantee a good outcome.

fetal position	胎児型姿勢
perforated	穿孔した，穴のある
admit	入院させる
chest pain	胸痛
localized	局部的な
surgery	手術
surgeon	外科医
outcome	結果，転帰

Notes (l. 1) be curled　からだを丸くする，丸くなって寝る　　(l. 1) back and forth　前後に，左右に
(l. 2) so ~ that ...　非常に~なので …　　(l. 3) on a 1-to-10 scale　1 からの 10 の 10 段階で
(l. 8) immediately　直ちに　　(l. 9) magnitude　大きさ　　(l. 10) work against ~　~に不利に働く

Check the situation

Q1 レイ・トロイアンの激痛の原因は？

Q2 レイ・トロイアンの手術を困難にしている 2 つの要因は？

Medical and Nursing Notes

under control　管理されて，抑制されて

　　　After Ray's pain was under better control, he lay stretched out on the bed, holding Kathryn's hand. They were deep in conversation, as if no one else in the world existed. There was no other family member to help them make this decision. I
5　left them alone while I checked on my other patients; when I returned to Ray's room, he told me that he and Kathryn decided there would be no surgery.

check on ~　～の様子を確認する

　　　He said it was an easy decision, and he was at peace with God. He'd lived a great life surrounded by the people he
10　loved, and he had no regrets. If it was his time, it was his time. Kathryn appeared calm, strong, and remarkably comfortable with this decision. Whenever I asked if either of them needed anything, she always declined, saying, "No, I'm fine, thanks." Once I shooed her out to take a short walk to stretch her legs.
15　She reluctantly went only after I promised to stay with Ray until she returned. I worried about her. I wasn't sure she understood what the next 24 hours would be like for her father.

　　　The most valuable care I could give him was comfort. These would be his last hours on earth, and I wanted to make
20　sure they were peaceful ones. I knew that as long as I kept his pain under control, Kathryn would be able to withstand the ending. After a few hours, Ray remained sleepy but alert. His condition worsened much faster than I'd anticipated, and although I was glad he wouldn't linger and suffer, I felt sad for
25　the short time he and Kathryn had left.

alert　頭が冴えて，機敏な

　　　When my 12-hour shift ended, I was asked to stay an additional four hours. Tired from such a busy day, I knew there was no one else to fill in. Ray deteriorated quickly; his

---

Notes

(l. 1) stretched out　手足を伸ばして　　　(l. 2) be deep in conversation　話し込んでいる
(l. 3) as if ~　まるで～であるかのように　　　(l. 8) at peace　心が安らいで
(l. 9) live a great life　素晴らしい人生を送る　　　(l. 11) remarkably　著しく　　　(l. 13) decline　断る
(l. 14) shoo　追い立てる　　　(l. 15) reluctantly　しぶしぶ　　　(l. 19) on earth　この世で
(l. 19) make sure ~　間違いなく～するようにする　　　(l. 20) as long as ~　～する限りは
(l. 21) be able to ~　～することができる　　　(l. 21) withstand　耐える，持ちこたえる
(l. 24) linger　生きながらえる　　　(l. 27) additional　追加の　　　(l. 28) fill in　代役を務める

vital signs fell, and his extremities became cold and mottled. He didn't respond to voice or touch. His lung sounds were coarse and audible without a stethoscope. He showed no outward signs of pain.

5   It had been just Ray and Kathryn for years now. Ray's wife, Wilma, had died from cancer three years before. It was a long, harrowing illness. They'd been married 57 years. By evening I felt close to Ray and Kathryn, like they were becoming a part of my own family. I told Kathryn I would be her father's nurse
10   until 11:30 PM. She seemed relieved.

      Shortly after 11 PM, Ray took his final breaths and was gone. Kathryn was there, telling him it was all right to go. He didn't fight his death; he let it consume him peacefully. It was only then that Kathryn cried. We stood at his bedside hugging.

15   I left Kathryn alone with her father. It was important that she have the time with him to say good-bye. When she was ready to go, she thanked me for all that I had done for her father, even though I had played such a small part in this once-vital man's last days. When I got home that night, I was at
20   peace with how that long day turned out. I, too, had no regrets.

Notes (l. 1) mottled　まだらの　　(l. 2) coarse　粗い　　(l. 3) audible　聞き取れる　　(l. 3) outward　外側から見た
(l. 7) harrowing　痛ましい　　(l. 10) relieved　ほっとした　　(l. 13) consume　使い尽くす
(l. 13) It is only then that ~　その時になって初めて~　　(l. 16) be ready to ~　~する準備ができている
(l. 18) even though ~　ではあるが　　(l. 18) once-vital　かつて生き生きしていた　　(l. 20) turn out ~　結局~となる

vital sign　（複数形で）バイタルサイン（呼吸数，脈拍数，体温，血圧など）
extremity　（複数形で）両手両足
lung　肺
stethoscope　聴診器

die from ~　~が原因で死ぬ
cancer　がん

take one's final breath　息を引き取る

Reading Comprehension

次の英文が，本文の内容と一致する場合は T，一致しない場合は F を選びなさい。

1. (T / F) Ray and Wilma decided not to have the surgery.
2. (T / F) Arlene (the writer) stayed with Ray while Kathryn was taking a short walk.
3. (T / F) Arlene tried to keep Ray's pain under control.
4. (T / F) Ray's wife died from cancer when she was 57 years old.
5. (T / F) When Ray died, Kathryn didn't cry at all.

Dictation & Translation `CD` `1-04` `▶` `04`

音声を聴いて英文の空欄に適語を記入しなさい。また，完成した英文を日本語に直しなさい。

1. She was walking _____ _____ _____ in the room.

   _____

2. It was difficult to keep my feelings _____ _____.

   _____

3. Could you _____ _____ for Mary while she's sick?

   _____

4. Are you _____ _____ go yet?

   _____

5. I still look fat, _____ _____ I've been exercising regularly.

   _____

Word Order & Translation `CD` `1-05` `▶` `05`

日本文の意味に合うように，（　）内の語句を並べかえて英文を作りなさい。

1. 我が家の子どもたちはとても疲れていたので，車の中で眠り込んでしまった。

   (were / they / the car / that / our children / asleep / so / in / fell / tired).

   _____

2. 私たちは健康的で幸せな暮らしを送る方法を学んだ。

   (life / and / live / learned / happy / to / healthy / how / we / a).

   _____

3. 問題点がない限りは，私たちはその仕事を金曜日までに終えられるはずだ。

   (we / Friday / are / should finish / long / by / as / no problems / there / as / the work).

   _____

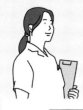

Nursing Terms and Expressions

次の日本文の空欄に入る語を下から選びなさい。

> うつ病， 関節炎， 心臓発作， 喘息， 糖尿病， 認知症， 脳卒中， 肺炎

1. My grandfather has **arthritis** in his knees.
   私の祖父は膝の＿＿＿＿＿＿＿を抱えている。

2. My sister suffers from **asthma** and must use an inhaler.
   私の妹は＿＿＿＿＿＿＿に苦しんでいるので， 吸入器を使わなければならない。

3. He has had **diabetes** since childhood but controls it with insulin.
   彼は子どもの時から＿＿＿＿＿＿＿だったが， インシュリンでコントロールしている。

4. The most common form of **dementia** is Alzheimer's disease.
   最もよくある種類の＿＿＿＿＿＿＿は， アルツハイマー病だ。

5. She suffered from **depression** after losing her job.
   仕事を失った後， 彼女は＿＿＿＿＿＿＿に苦しんだ。

6. She had a mild **heart attack** but won't need an operation.
   彼女は軽い＿＿＿＿＿＿＿を起こしたが， 手術は必要ないだろう。

7. My grandmother nearly died of **pneumonia**.
   私の祖母は＿＿＿＿＿＿＿で死ぬところだった。

8. I looked after my mother after she had a **stroke**.
   母が＿＿＿＿＿＿＿を起こした後， 私は母の世話をした。

Column

世界的な糖尿病の脅威に対して 1991 年に制定されたのが World Diabetes Day（世界糖尿病デー）です。2006 年には国連によって正式に認められました。インスリン（insulin）を発見した Sir Frederick Banting の誕生日である 11 月 14 日が， この World Diabetes Day となっています。

さて， この diabetes という語をまだ知らない， 小児糖尿病で入院中の女の子が， 自分の余命が長くないと勘違いしてしまったというエピソードがあります。その子の耳には， diabetes が "die of beeties"（「beeties が原因で死ぬ」）と聞こえていたのです。もちろん， "beeties" という名前の病気はありません。

Unit 2
Ordinary Things

What gets you through the night shift?
*get A thorough B　A に B を切り抜けさせる

Cindy McCoy, PhD, MSN, RN-BC

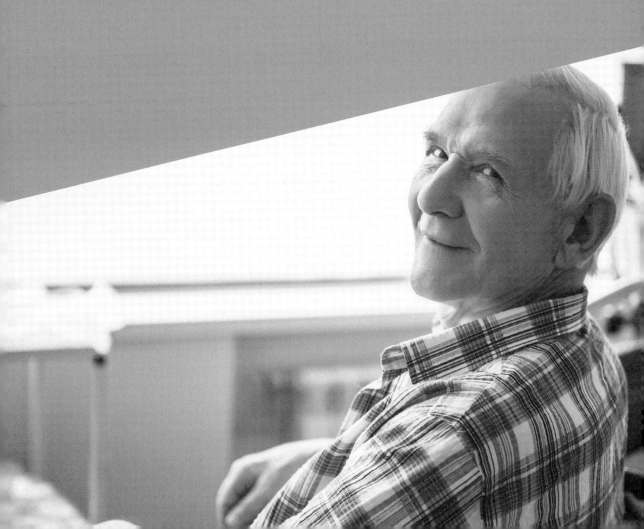

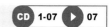

次の英語の意味に合う日本語を下から選びなさい。また，音声を聴いて発音しなさい。

1. defibrillator _____ **2.** catheter _____

3. ventilator _____ **4.** infection _____

5. tolerate _____

人工呼吸器，カテーテル，我慢する，除細動器，感染症

READING **Essay【Part 1】** CD 1-07 ▶ 07

エッセイの出だしを読んでみましょう。

Medical and Nursing Notes

　　　Carol's patient is in ventricular tachycardia again. In her 70s, the patient's been without brain function since she went into cardiac arrest while singing in her church choir. When I hear Carol call to me, I raise the side rail on my patient's bed, hurry
5　across the cardiac ICU, and snatch the crash cart. As I shove it close to the bedside, Carol grabs the defibrillator paddles and shocks the patient. When the monitor shows no change in rhythm, Carol delivers another shock. This time it works; we watch for a minute to make sure the rhythm continues, then
10　Carol goes to call the physician while I check the patient's IV, endotracheal tube, and urinary catheter.

　　　We're understaffed, with six patients between us. Sometimes, at the start of a night shift, it's hard to feel positive when you know it might not be possible to provide the best care.
15　We're several hours into the shift now, and saving this patient's life feels good. When Carol returns with her orders, we quickly prepare the medication and the new IV infusion.

ventricular tachycardia	心室性頻拍
brain	脳
cardiac arrest	心拍停止
cardiac ICU	心臓疾患集中治療室（cardiac intensive care unit）
crash cart	クラッシュカート（患者が「クラッシュ」つまり，心拍停止状態になった時に治療するための医療器具などを運ぶカート）
paddle	電極
shock	電気ショックを与える
rhythm	心律動（cardiac rhythm）
IV	点滴（intravenous）
endotracheal tube	気管内チューブ
urinary	尿の
night shift	夜勤
medication	投薬
infusion	輸液剤

Notes (l. 3) choir 聖歌隊　　(l. 4) call to ~ 〜を大声で呼ぶ　　(l. 5) snatch ひっつかむ　　(l. 5) shove 乱暴に押す
(l. 8) deliver 与える　　(l. 9) make sure ~ 間違いなく〜するようにする　　(l. 12) understaffed 人手不足の

Check the situation

Q1 キャロル担当の患者は何をしている時に心拍停止になったか？

Q2 夜勤が始まる時にシンディ（筆者）が前向きな気持ちになれないのはどんな場合か？

Medical and Nursing Notes

make a round　巡回する

I return to my patient, who has dozed off, then make a hasty round of the other patients: an IV bag needs to be replaced, a patient needs assistance onto a bedpan, another needs to be repositioned.

IV bag　点滴バッグ，輸液バッグ

bedpan　便器

reposition　体位を変える

5　Since Carol's patient seems to have stabilized, I make a trip to the waiting room outside the unit. As I open the door several sets of sleepy eyes question me. I always dread this part of the job. No one wants me to call her or his name. I beckon the patient's daughter to the door, quietly explain the event, 10　and ask her if she'd like to come in and talk to her mother. She smiles and follows me onto the unit. Even though her mother is sedated and on a ventilator, the daughter stands and talks to her, stroking her hair, holding her hand. I leave as Carol comes in to speak with the daughter.

stabilize　安定する

sedate　（鎮静剤で）眠らせる

15　My total-care ventilator patient needs a bath. I've cared for him every night for two weeks. In his early 60s, he crashed his car after a myocardial infarction. Since then he's had heart failure and acute respiratory distress syndrome and now has an abdominal dressing because of an infection at the site of an 20　exploratory laparoscopy.

total-care　トータルケアの（身体的・精神的ケア，患者・家族のケアなど全てを含む）
bath　清拭（bed bath）
care for ~　~の世話をする
myocardial infarction　心筋梗塞
heart failure　心不全
acute respiratory distress syndrome　急性呼吸窮迫症候群
abdominal dressing　腹部（開放創用）ドレッシング（dressing は創傷被覆材のこと）
exploratory laparoscopy　試験開腹術

I can tell from his expression that he's depressed. Some of the other nurses don't like to work with him because he can be irritable if you do things for him without telling him first. I figured this out early and we get along fine. He's awake and 25　alert and communicates well—mouthing words and using hand gestures—even with his tracheotomy tube. He likes to watch country music videos; we turn the TV on and I sing along. As I perform tracheotomy care and change his abdominal dressing, I talk to him about his family, their pets. After I bathe him, he 30　and I decide that we will try sitting him up in the chair for a

alert　機敏な

tracheotomy tube　気管切開チューブ

bathe　清拭する

Notes

(l. 1) doze off　うとうと眠り込む　　(l. 2) hasty　急いだ　　(l. 5) seem to ~　~のように思われる
(l. 7) dread　ひどく怖がる　　(l. 8) beckon　（身振りなどで）招く　　(l. 10) 'd like to ~　~したいと思う（would like to ~）
(l. 11) even though ~　~ではあるが　　(l. 13) stroke　なでる　　(l. 19) because of ~　~が原因で
(l. 21) depressed　意気消沈した，ふさぎ込んだ　　(l. 22) work with ~　~のために働く，~を相手に働く
(l. 23) irritable　怒りっぽい　　(l. 24) figure ~ out　~を理解する　　(l. 24) get along　仲良くやっていく
(l. 25) mouth　（声に出さずに）口の動きで伝える　　(l. 27) turn ~ on　（スイッチを押して）~をつける
(l. 27) sing along　一緒に歌う　　(l. 30) for a while　しばらくの間

while. His wife usually comes in at about 6:30 AM, and we plan to surprise her. Carol and I enlist the help of the respiratory therapist, and together we help him up into the chair at the bedside. Although I have much to accomplish before the end

5 of my shift, I decide to wash his hair and shave him. When he is clean, groomed, and smiling, we prop him up. He seems to tolerate it well.

respiratory therapist　呼吸療法士

The sun starts to come in through the windows. Carol makes a fresh pot of coffee. There's still a bag of dirty linens to

10 empty, a drug cart to be exchanged, the schedule to review, and the crash cart to be restocked.

drug cart　与薬カート

My patient's wife peeks around the unit's door at 6:30. Visiting hours don't begin until 9, but I always let her in early. I tell her we have a surprise for her. As she enters her husband's

visiting hours　面会時間

15 room, I watch from outside the door. His smile matches hers. I give them a few minutes, then go in. "Thank you so much," she says. She is crying. "He is going to be okay. I know it now. He looks like himself today."

I ask him if he'd like to go back to bed, but he says no. I

20 leave them together holding hands.

Since I became a full-time teacher, it's moments like these that I miss the most—even more, maybe, than saving lives.

Notes　(l. 2) enlist　得る　　(l. 4) accomplish　成し遂げる　　(l. 6) groom　身づくろいする　　(l. 6) prop ~ up　～をもたせかける
(l. 10) empty　取り去る　　(l. 11) restock　補充する　　(l. 12) peek　こっそりのぞく　　(l. 13) let ~ in　～を中に入れる
(l. 21) it's A that ~　～なのは A である

Reading Comprehension

次の英文が，本文の内容と一致する場合は T，一致しない場合は F を選びなさい。

1. (T / F) One of Cindy's patients began to sleep, so she made her rounds of the other patients in a hurry.

2. (T / F) Cindy's total-care patient suffered from myocardial infarction while singing in his church choir.

3. (T / F) Cindy's patient got along well with the other nurses.

4. (T / F) When the day was beginning to break, Cindy and Carol had a drug cart to be changed and a crash cart to be restocked.

5. (T / F) Cindy always let the patient's wife in before visiting hours began.

音声を聴いて英文の空欄に適語を記入しなさい。また，完成した英文を日本語に直しなさい。

1. Tom _____ _____ watching TV.

   _____

2. I _____ _____ _____ go abroad next year.

   _____

3. She's _____ _____ children who have learning difficulties.

   _____

4. They seem to be _____ _____ much better these days.

   _____

5. I haven't seen him _____ _____ _____.

   _____

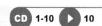

日本文の意味に合うように，（　）内の語句を並べかえて英文を作りなさい。

1. 間違いなく車がロックされているようにします。

   (the car / sure / is / that / make / locked / I'll).

   _____

2. 雨だったので私たちは散歩に行かなかった。

   (the rain / because / for / didn't / of / a walk / go / we).

   _____

3. 彼らがオーストラリアへ行ったのは去年のことだ。

   (Australia / it / to / was / went / last year / they / that).

   _____

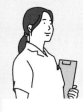

Nursing Terms and Expressions

次の英文の空欄に入る語を下から選びなさい。また，その英文に合う写真の記号を [ ] 内に入れなさい。

---

bedpan,   endoscope,   forceps,   stethoscope,   urinal,   ventilator,   wheelchair

---

1. Take the covered _____ to the utility room and observe its contents. [   ]
   蓋のついた**便器**をユーティリティールームに持って行って，中身を観察しなさい。

2. Surgeons use _____ during surgical procedures to hold onto tissues and to clamp blood vessels. [   ]
   外科医は，外科的処置の際に，組織をつかんだり血管をクランプしたりするために**鉗子**を使う。

3. The doctor listened to the patient's heart with his _____ for 3 minutes. [   ]
   その医師は，**聴診器**でその患者の胸の音を3分間聴いた。

4. A _____ is a container used to collect urine. [   ]
   尿瓶は，尿を集めるのに使われる容器だ。

5. The patient was put on a _____ but died three hours later. [   ]
   その患者は**人工呼吸器**につながれたが，3時間後に死亡した。

6. The nurse pushed the sick child in a _____. [   ]
   その看護師は，**車椅子**に乗せてその病気の子どもを押した。

7. An _____ can be used to look into the esophagus, stomach, duodenum, colon, rectum, or other organs. [   ]
   内視鏡は，食道，胃，十二指腸，結腸，直腸，その他の臓器の中を見るために使うことができる。

ア　　　　　　　イ　　　　　　　ウ　　　　　　　エ

オ　　　　　　　カ　　　　　　　キ

Unit 3
Making It Fit

*A new NP on a psych unit finds
her professional identity must be redefined.*
* redefine　見直す

Meredith Bailey, MSN, BSN, RN, PMH-NP

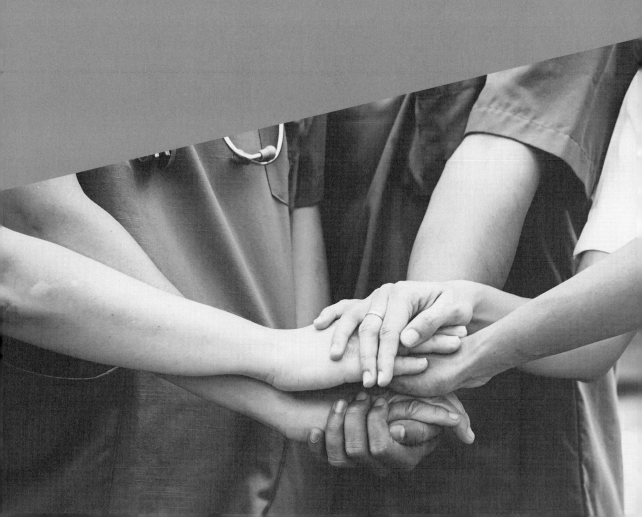

次の英語の意味に合う日本語を下から選びなさい。また，音声を聴いて発音しなさい。

1. treatment _____

2. psychiatrist _____

3. pediatric _____

4. chaos _____

5. seizure _____

大混乱，小児科の，精神科医，発作，治療

READING **Essay【Part 1】** CD 1-12 ▶ 12

エッセイの出だしを読んでみましょう。

Medical and Nursing Notes

I work on an inpatient psychiatric unit and introduce myself as an advanced practice nurse or an NP. Often, patients look at me curiously and respond with something like, "So you're the head nurse?" Then I explain that no, I'm not the head nurse. I'm
5　in charge of their treatment plan, medications, and discharge planning. This is followed by, "So you're like a doctor?"

　　Most of the time, I sigh and say yes, I suppose I'm kind of like a doctor. But my whole being rebels at defining my nursing practice as "like a doctor." I'm not a doctor. I'm a nurse. In my
10　newest nursing role, it's been challenging to be trained by a psychiatrist and not initially welcomed by nursing colleagues. When I walked onto the unit my first day, expecting to be embraced by the nurses, I was dumbfounded and hurt that my own profession didn't accept me with open arms. The inpatient
15　unit is a melting pot of professions, and I found that I didn't necessarily fit with the doctors, the social workers, or the staff nurses.

inpatient　入院患者（の）
psychiatric unit　精神科病棟
advanced practice nurse　高度実践看護師（APN）
NP　ナースプラクティショナー（nurse practitioner）
head nurse　看護師長

in charge of ~　~を担当して
treatment　治療
medication　投薬
discharge　退院

social worker　ソーシャルワーカー
staff nurse　ベッドサイドでケアを行う登録看護師（registered nurse）で，bedside nurse, clinical nurse, floor nurse とほぼ同義

Notes
(l. 7) most of the time　ほとんどの場合は　　(l. 7) kind of ~　多少~　　(l. 8) whole being　からだ全体
(l. 8) rebel at ~　~に反感を持つ　　(l. 8) define A as B　A を B と定義する，A を B と考える
(l. 13) embrace　抱きしめる　　(l. 13) dumbfound　唖然とさせる　　(l. 14) with open arms　両手を広げて，心から
(l. 15) melting pot　るつぼ　　(l. 15) not necessarily ~　必ずしも~とは限らない

Check the situation

Q1 メレディス（筆者）が精神科の入院患者に対して担当したこと 3 つは何か？

Q2 当初メレディスが必ずしもうまく馴染めなかったスタッフは？

Medical and Nursing Notes

APRN 高度実践登録看護師
（advanced practice registered nurse)
ED 救急部門 （emergency
department)

I was a new APRN, but I'd worked as a staff nurse in a pediatric ED for six years. I had been through a lot in the ED, personally and professionally. I'd come to consider my nurse colleagues as friends and teammates. We had each other's backs
5　through the best and worst of times. In the chaos of an ED, it's imperative that the nurses unite, and we did. I'd assumed that this feeling of being a team carried across departments, hospitals, and roles.

　I was wrong. There were staff meetings for nurses only
10　and I wasn't invited. I was expected to go to medical staff meetings weekly—except on the weeks when the meetings were physicians only. I received a message, loud and clear, that I was something different, and I didn't like it.

　I didn't experience nurses "eating their young." It was
15　worse—they ignored me. At first I cried. I left each night feeling like I'd made a mistake in leaving the ED and entering this new role. I didn't want to be an APRN. I wanted to go back to being an RN. I felt like everything was backward. I now had residents and medical students following me around and doing rounds
20　with me. My only experience with residents up to that point had been in the ED, and certainly not in a supervisory role.

RN 登録看護師 （registered nurse)
resident 研修医
do rounds 巡回する

　It took time and a lot of patience, but eventually I started to accept and engage with my new role. The attending I work with is a psychiatrist and we often have nurse versus doctor
25　debates. He helps me become an independent practitioner and I help him be more like a nurse. He also helps me navigate the challenges presented by my patients, the unit, and the hospital.

attending 在籍医師, 指導医, 主
治医 （attending physician)

　The medical consulting APRN also befriended me, and after my first month I told her my worry that the other nurses
30　didn't accept me. She bluntly told me I wasn't a staff nurse

Notes
(l. 2) be through ~ 　～を経験して 　　(l. 4) have A's back 　A を守る，A を助ける
(l. 6) imperative 　必須の，避けられない 　　(l. 6) unite 　団結する 　　(l. 7) carry across ~ 　～に届く
(l. 12) loud and clear 　非常に明瞭に
(l. 14) eat one's young 　自分よりも下の地位や立場のメンバーを無視したり，裏切ったり，厳しく非難したりする
(l. 15) at first 　最初は 　　(l. 18) backward 　後退して，悪い状態で 　　(l. 20) up to ~ 　～に至るまで
(l. 21) supervisory 　監督の，管理の 　　(l. 23) engage with ~ 　～になじむ，～をかみ合う
(l. 26) navigate 　切り抜ける 　　(l. 28) consulting 　助言を与える 　　(l. 28) befriend 　味方となる，助ける
(l. 30) bluntly 　ぶっきらぼうに 　　(l. 30) not ~ anymore 　もはや～ではない

anymore, so I should buck up and things would get better. That felt like nurse advice, and I didn't feel so alone any longer. Realizing that I couldn't be the only person experiencing this, I started to organize a meeting of all the psychiatric APRNs at

5 the institution.

During my second month, some of the nurses realized that I could put medication and diet orders in and that I'm more accessible than my attending, so a few started speaking to me. During my third month, there was a seizure on the unit and I

10 was the only provider on the floor. I handled myself well, and after that all the nurses began talking to me. I have done blood draws on hard sticks on the unit, and I drop by electroconvulsive therapy three times a week to place ivs so I can keep my skills up. It took time and energy, but I proved that I'm not scared to

15 get my hands dirty and I'm definitely not "like a doctor."

After six months, a few of the nurses invited me to dinner. I immediately accepted, and while we were having our meal we talked about the difficulties they'd had with me and I'd had with them. We laughed because it seemed silly now, but in the

20 beginning they didn't know where I fit into their world and I didn't know where they fit into mine. But I knew I was going to make them fit—because, like I said, in my heart and in my practice, I'm a nurse.

provider （医療）提供者

blood draw　採血

hard stick　採血しにくい患者
（tough stick とも呼ばれる）
electroconvulsive therapy　電気痙
攣療法（ECT）
iv　静脈点滴（intravenous）

Notes (l. 1) buck up　元気を出す　　(l. 2) not ~ any longer　もはや〜ではない　　(l. 4) organize　取りまとめる
(l. 8) accessible　近づきやすい，つきあいやすい　　(l. 10) handle oneself　ふるまう
(l. 12) drop by ~　〜に立ち寄る　　(l. 14) be scared to ~　〜することを怖がって
(l. 15) get one's hands dirty　肉体労働をする　　(l. 19) in the beginning　まず最初は　　(l. 20) fit into ~　〜になじむ

Reading Comprehension

次の英文が，本文の内容と一致する場合は T，一致しない場合は F を選びなさい。

1. (T / F)　Meredith had worked as a staff nurse in a pediatric clinic for six years.

2. (T / F)　Meredith wasn't invited to nursing staff meetings, but she could go to staff meetings for physicians.

3. (T / F)　The attending psychiatrist helped Meredith navigate the challenges in the hospital.

4. (T / F)　All the nurses began to talk to Meredith during her second month.

5. (T / F)　Half a year later, Meredith was accepted and some nurses invited her to dinner.

音声を聴いて英文の空欄に適語を記入しなさい。また，完成した英文を日本語に直しなさい。

1. It's ＿＿＿＿＿＿＿＿＿ ＿＿＿＿＿＿＿＿＿ dark in here.

＿＿＿＿＿＿＿＿＿＿＿＿＿＿＿＿＿＿＿＿＿＿＿＿＿＿＿＿＿＿＿＿＿＿＿

2. We welcomed her ＿＿＿＿＿＿＿＿＿ ＿＿＿＿＿＿＿＿＿ ＿＿＿＿＿＿＿＿＿.

＿＿＿＿＿＿＿＿＿＿＿＿＿＿＿＿＿＿＿＿＿＿＿＿＿＿＿＿＿＿＿＿＿＿＿

3. The message was ＿＿＿＿＿＿＿＿＿ ＿＿＿＿＿＿＿＿＿ ＿＿＿＿＿＿＿＿＿.

＿＿＿＿＿＿＿＿＿＿＿＿＿＿＿＿＿＿＿＿＿＿＿＿＿＿＿＿＿＿＿＿＿＿＿

4. ＿＿＿＿＿＿＿＿＿ ＿＿＿＿＿＿＿＿＿ now, she's been very quiet.

＿＿＿＿＿＿＿＿＿＿＿＿＿＿＿＿＿＿＿＿＿＿＿＿＿＿＿＿＿＿＿＿＿＿＿

5. She didn't take me seriously ＿＿＿＿＿＿＿＿＿ ＿＿＿＿＿＿＿＿＿ ＿＿＿＿＿＿＿＿＿.

＿＿＿＿＿＿＿＿＿＿＿＿＿＿＿＿＿＿＿＿＿＿＿＿＿＿＿＿＿＿＿＿＿＿＿

日本文の意味に合うように，（ ）内の語句を並べかえて英文を作りなさい。

1. この場所はほとんどの場合は本当に混雑している。

(the time / most / really / this place / of / busy / is).

＿＿＿＿＿＿＿＿＿＿＿＿＿＿＿＿＿＿＿＿＿＿＿＿＿＿＿＿＿＿＿＿＿＿＿

2. 君は必ずしもそのパーティーに行く必要はない。

(don't / the party / have / go / you / to / necessarily / to).

＿＿＿＿＿＿＿＿＿＿＿＿＿＿＿＿＿＿＿＿＿＿＿＿＿＿＿＿＿＿＿＿＿＿＿

3. 彼はもはやその会社で働いていない。

(longer / he / any / does / the company / not / for / work).

＿＿＿＿＿＿＿＿＿＿＿＿＿＿＿＿＿＿＿＿＿＿＿＿＿＿＿＿＿＿＿＿＿＿＿

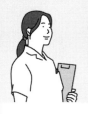

LEARN MORE

Nursing Terms and Expressions

診療科について，次の表の（　）内に入る語を下から選びなさい。

English	definition	Japanese
internal medicine	a branch of medicine concerned with the treatment of diseases without doing medical operations	内科
surgery	a branch of medicine concerned with treating diseases or injuries by means of manual or operative procedures	外科
pediatrics	a branch of medicine that deals with [1].(　　　　　　) and their diseases	小児科
obstetrics	a branch of medicine that deals with [2].(　　　　　　) and the birth of babies	産科
gynecology	a branch of medicine that deals with the diseases and routine physical care of the reproductive system of women	5. (　　　　)
orthopedics	a branch of medicine that deals with injuries and diseases of the bones or muscles	6. (　　　　)
psychiatry	a branch of medicine that deals with mental, emotional, or behavioral disorders	7. (　　　　)
dermatology	a branch of medicine dealing with the [3].(　　　　), its structure, functions, and diseases	皮膚科
ophthalmology	a branch of medical science dealing with the structure, functions, and diseases of the eye	眼科
radiology	a branch of medicine concerned with the use of radiation, especially [4].(　　　　　　)	放射線科
urology	a branch of medicine concerned with the parts of the body that produce and carry urine	8. (　　　　)

skin, children, X-rays, pregnancy	整形外科，精神科，泌尿器科，婦人科

Column

　接尾辞（suffix）の -ian や -ist は，「～を専門とする人」の意味の単語を形成します。例えば，pediatrics なら pediatrician（小児科医），gynecology なら gynecologist（婦人科医），psychiatrics なら psychiatrist（精神科医）となります。

　ところで，スラングでは surgeon（外科医）を knife-happy と呼ぶことがあります。「やたらに引金（trigger）を引きたがる」という意味の trigger-happy に倣って，「やたらに knife（メス）を使って手術をしたがる（外科医）」ということです。それに対して，internist（内科医）を flea と呼ぶことがあります。患者にべったりとくっついて離れない様子を flea（ノミ）に喩えたという説があります。

　次の語が指している医師を下から選んで日本語に直してみましょう。

1. baby catcher（赤ちゃんをキャッチする人）　　2. carpenter（大工）　　3. gas passer（ガスを送る人）

4. neuron（神経単位）　　5. shadow gazer（影を見つめる人）

anesthesiologist, neurologist, obstetrician, orthopedist, radiologist

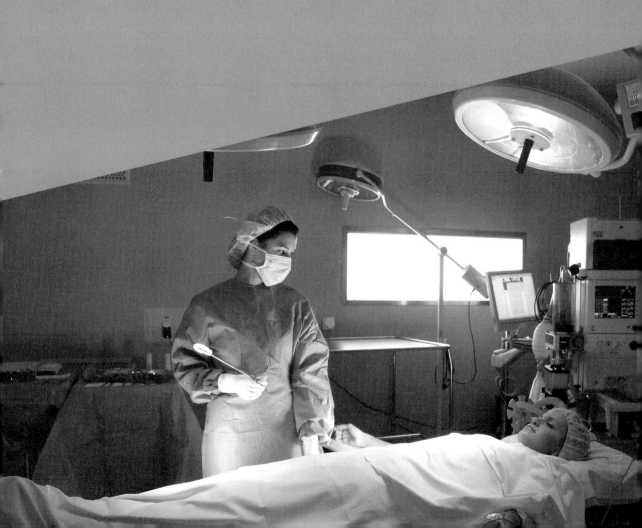

Unit 4
Promises to Keep

A 'routine' organ harvesting and a family's request.

Judy Morse, ASN, RN

次の英語の意味に合う日本語を下から選びなさい。また，音声を聴いて発音しなさい。

1. procurement ＿＿＿＿＿＿＿＿

2. anesthesiologist ＿＿＿＿＿＿＿＿

3. reassure ＿＿＿＿＿＿＿＿

4. suture ＿＿＿＿＿＿＿＿

5. morgue ＿＿＿＿＿＿＿＿

> 安心させる，麻酔専門医，遺体安置所，調達，縫合

READING **Essay【Part 1】**　CD 1-17 ▶ 17

エッセイの出だしを読んでみましょう。

Medical and Nursing Notes

"You have a harvesting for a patient in the ICU," said the voice on the other end of the line. It was Saturday, I was on call, and my morning routine—laundry, housecleaning—was officially over. This was to be my first organ procurement. I got

5　in my car and began the 15-minute drive to the hospital. I had some idea about my role, but was unsure about specifics: What instruments would I need? Where would I get the ice? How long would it take? How would the family react?

　　Soon after arriving at the hospital, I began to prepare the

10　operating room with Ruth. She and I had worked together since I began on the unit three years before. She was very experienced, which gave me some comfort, especially on call. I counted on Ruth to get me through.

harvesting　臓器摘出（organ harvesting）
ICU　集中治療室（intensive care unit）
on call　待機して，当直で

organ　臓器

operating room　手術室

Notes　(l. 3) be over　終わって　　(l. 6) be unsure about ~　~に自信がない　　(l. 6) specific　（複数形で）詳細
(l. 13) count on A to ~　~することを A に頼る　　(l. 13) get A through　A を乗り越えさせる

Check the situation

　Q1　土曜日の朝，ジュディ（筆者）にかかってきた電話の内容は？

　Q2　ジュディとルースの関係は？

Medical and Nursing Notes

　　As we gathered instruments and supplies, Elizabeth, the transplantation coordinator, came to brief us on the patient, a 45-year-old woman named Lynne who had brain death following a stroke. Her briefing was just that—brief—before she
5　returned to the family.

　　When the transplantation team was ready, Elizabeth came to let us know. Ruth, the anesthesiologist, and I followed her to Lynne's room in the ICU. Family and friends surrounded her bed, visibly shaken, mourning the death that was to come.
10　Some were crying, others were hugging, and one elderly woman sat quietly in the corner. I was unsure about what would happen next. Would the family leave before we wheeled Lynne to the operating room? Would they follow, as other families did? How could I walk over to the bed, unlock the wheels, and
15　push the patient to the operating room as I had done so many times before? This time, there would be no return. I could not reassure Lynne's family that we would take excellent care of her.

　　Elizabeth introduced me to Lynne's sister. Instead of shaking her hand, I touched her arm. The three of us walked
20　toward Lynne's bed, and Elizabeth told me of the family's request that Lynne not be left alone at any time. Her sister handed me a neatly folded pile of clothing—underwear; plain, dark slacks; and a long-sleeved, striped T-shirt—and asked that I dress Lynne after we were done. That's all they wanted.

25　Lynne's family stayed behind as we wheeled her out of the ICU.

　　In the operating room, I fell into my usual routine. Tending to the patient, keeping things in order, assisting the anesthesiologist, documenting—these were all tasks I had
30　done many times before. As each procedure was completed,

Medical and Nursing Notes

transplantation coordinator　臓器移植コーディネーター
brain death　脳死

stroke　脳卒中

transplantation team　臓器移植チーム

wheel　（ストレッチャーなどで）運ぶ

take care of ~　～の世話をする

tend to ~　～の世話をする

Notes　(l. 2) brief　要点を話す　　(l. 9) visibly　明らかに　　(l. 9) shaken　動揺して　　(l. 9) mourn　嘆き悲しむ
(l. 10) some ~ others ...　～もいれば，…もいる　　(l. 18) instead of ~　～する代わりに
(l. 21) at any time　どんな時でも　　(l. 22) a pile of ~　山のような～　　(l. 22) neatly　きちんと
(l. 22) folded　折りたたんだ　　(l. 27) fall into ~　～を始める　　(l. 28) keep ~ in order　～を整理しておく

the team grew smaller. Within two hours, Lynne's liver had been removed, the sutures were in place, life-support had been withdrawn, the medical team had gone, and Ruth had left to clean the instruments. I was suddenly alone with Lynne.

5　How little I knew of this woman. But there were tasks still to be done. I needed towels, warm water, and soap. I set out to retrieve them. At the door, I stopped and looked back. Lynne's body was exposed, alone in the big, empty room. I remembered her family's request. Returning to her bedside, I covered Lynne
10　with a blanket, sat down on a stool beside her, and waited for Ruth.

Ruth returned about five minutes later. Noticing that the body and the room remained unchanged, she looked surprised. "I was waiting for you," I said. "We can't leave her alone." She
15　smiled. Together we cleansed and dressed Lynne, then brought her to the morgue.

Outside the operating suite, Lynne's sister was standing in the hallway. She was alone. Without a word, she looked me in the eyes. I gave her a nod. She returned my nod, turned, and
20　walked away.

liver　肝臓

life-support　生命維持，延命処置

operating suite　手術室

Notes　(l. 2) in place　適切で　　(l. 3) withdraw　打ち切る　　(l. 6) set out to ~　～しはじめる　　(l. 15) cleanse　洗い清める
(l. 18) hallway　廊下　　(l. 18) look A in the eye(s)　A をまともに見る　　(l. 19) give A a nod　A に会釈をする

Reading Comprehension

次の英文が，本文の内容と一致する場合は T，一致しない場合は F を選びなさい。

1. (T / F) The transplantation coordinator briefly explained about the organ donor.
2. (T / F) When Ruth and Judy went into Lynne's room in the ICU, she had already died.
3. (T / F) In the operating room, the transplant team removed Lynne's lung within two hours.
4. (T / F) Elizabeth and Judy cleaned and dressed Lynne and brought her to the morgue.
5. (T / F) Lynne's sister said nothing, but she thanked Judy for not leaving Lynne alone.

音声を聴いて英文の空欄に適語を記入しなさい。また，完成した英文を日本語に直しなさい。

1. Dr. Greene will be _____ _____ this weekend.

_____

2. They became friends when the war _____ _____.

_____

3. Smoking is not allowed _____ _____ _____.

_____

4. I have _____ _____ _____ work to do today.

_____

5. Look me _____ _____ _____ and tell me you're not lying.

_____

日本文の意味に合うように，（　）内の語句を並べかえて英文を作りなさい。

1. すぐに大きくなる腫瘍もあれば，ゆっくり大きくなるものもある。
(quickly / grow / others / tumors / slowly / grow / some).

_____

2. 私たちは車ではなく電車で行った。
(by / went / of / we / by / instead / train / car).

_____

3. 物事を整頓しておくことが得意ですか?
(you / order / keeping / good / are / in / things / at)?

_____

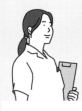

Nursing Terms and Expressions

次の日本文の空欄に入る語を下から選びなさい。

移植，　化学療法，　浣腸，　吸引，　挿管，　透析，　縫合，　輸血

---

1. Doctors often recommend **chemotherapy** as a treatment for cancer.
   医師は，しばしばがんの治療として＿＿＿＿＿＿＿を勧める。

2. She has been on **dialysis** three times a week.
   彼女は週 3 回＿＿＿＿＿＿＿を受けてきた。

3. The nurse gave the patient an **enema** before the operation.
   看護師は，手術前その患者に＿＿＿＿＿＿＿をした。

4. The opposite of **intubation** is extubation.
   ＿＿＿＿＿＿＿の反対は抜管だ。

5. A **suction** catheter is a medical device used to extract bodily secretions.
   ＿＿＿＿＿＿＿カテーテルは，体分泌物を取り除くために使われる医療機器だ。

6. **Sutures** are the most commonly used means of wound closure.
   ＿＿＿＿＿＿＿は，創傷閉鎖で最もよく使われる方法だ。

7. Most fatal **transfusion** reactions result from human error.
   ほとんどの致命的な＿＿＿＿＿＿＿副作用は，ヒューマンエラーが原因だ。

8. Organ **transplantation** is one of the great advances in modern medicine.
   臓器＿＿＿＿＿＿＿は，現代医療における大きな進歩のひとつだ。

Column

　英語の略語のなかに「切り株語」（stump word）と呼ばれるものがあります。例えば，chemotherapy → chemo, ventilator → vent, doctor → doc のように単語の頭部を残した型が最も多いです。カタカナ語で「リハビリテーション」→「リハビリ」ですが，英語では rehabilitation → rehab です。次に多いのは，telephone → phone のように単語の尾部を残した型で，influenza → flu のように単語の頭部と尾部を省略した型はとてもまれです。

Unit 5

The Eyes of a Pediatric Nurse

Could lessons learned from children apply to adults?

* apply to ~ 　〜に当てはまる

Beverly Rossiter, MSN, CRNP, CPNP

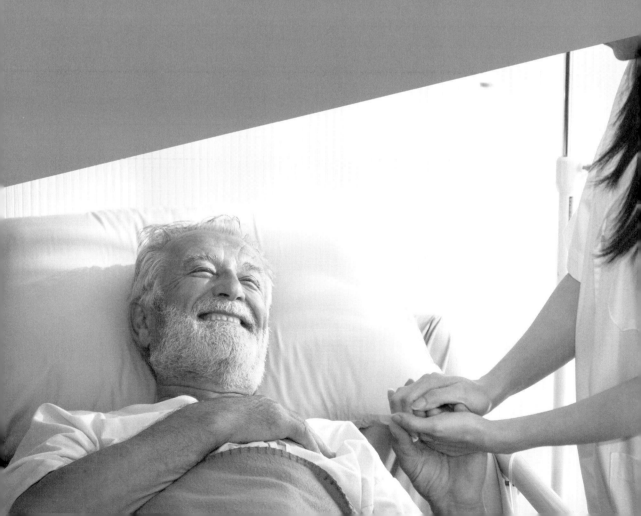

次の英語の意味に合う日本語を下から選びなさい。また，音声を聴いて発音しなさい。

1. demeanor 　　_____
2. admission 　　_____
3. pneumonia 　　_____
4. temperament 　　_____
5. cane 　　_____

気質，杖，態度，肺炎，入院

READING　　**Essay【Part 1】**　　CD 1-22 ▶ 22

エッセイの出だしを読んでみましょう。

Medical and Nursing Notes

Slowly, quietly, I entered 85-year-old Ronald Dixon's room. I was nervous. After 24 years as a pediatric nurse, I was seeing my first adult patient. As a professional, I knew the cries of a hurting baby, the stoic demeanor of the frightened school-age
5　child, the need to put "Dolly" in a toddler's surgical bed as she headed to the operating room. But would I achieve the same understanding with my adult patients? Before starting this new job, I asked myself: Would what I knew about caring for children be of any use with adults?
10　　As an admissions nurse, I didn't have to rush, and by habit I entered slowly and spoke softly. *Fast movement and speech can be frightening.* Mr. Dixon's reaction was my immediate reward—mirroring my relaxed demeanor, his dark eyes shone with warmth under a shock of bright white hair. Although
15　frail in his white and blue hospital gown, his welcome was hearty. He introduced me to his daughter, Margaret, and his granddaughter Vicki. I shook hands all around.

pediatric　小児科の

surgical bed　外科用ベッド
operating room　手術室

care for ~　～の世話をする

hospital gown　病衣

Notes
(l. 4) stoic　我慢強い　　(l. 5) "Dolly"　ぬいぐるみの「ドリー」　　(l. 5) toddler　よちよち歩きの幼児
(l. 9) of use　役に立って（useful）　　(l. 10) by habit　習慣で　　(l. 12) frightening　怖い　　(l. 12) immediate　すぐの
(l. 14) a shock of hair　くしゃくしゃの髪　　(l. 15) frail　弱々しい　　(l. 15) welcome　反応　　(l. 16) hearty　心からの
(l. 17) shake hands all around　握手をして回る

Check the situation

Q1　ビバリー（筆者）がディクソンの病室で不安だった理由は？
Q2　ディクソンはどのようにしてビバリーを温かく迎えてくれたか？

Medical and Nursing Notes

Pulling a chair to the head of Mr. Dixon's bed, I sat down and looked into his eyes. *Standing over a patient can be authoritative or frightening.* He had chronic obstructive pulmonary disease and had been admitted from the ED with pneumonia. "I read the

5　ED report," I told him. "It sure sounds like you've had some struggles. Why don't you tell me how you've been feeling?" As Mr. Dixon explained his medical condition, I touched his hand. *Show them you are not running away.* His speech slowed and his story gained clarity. He told me about his wife, who'd died only

10　three years prior. They'd been married nearly 50 years. She had cancer, and he was her caretaker until the end. As he related the story he averted his eyes; I did the same. *Mirror the patient's tempo and temperament to establish rapport.*

I then turned my attention to Margaret and Vicki, who

15　were standing at his bedside. Margaret was obviously troubled; she'd crossed her arms tightly and her hands were tugging on the elbows of her silk blouse. *Who else in the room is in need?* "It sounds like you've been having a rough time. You must have been really scared when his breathing trouble started."

20　Margaret described difficulties at work and problems with getting her dad to doctor's appointments. "His breathing's been bad, and it's getting worse. We don't know what to do anymore," she admitted. "You're doing the right thing," I reassured her. "Is there anything special that we should

25　know to ensure your dad gets the best care?" *Family can provide invaluable insight into the patient.* We discussed his tendency to get out of bed at night without using his cane. She was comforted when she found that the bed alarm would ring if he was to

---

chronic obstructive pulmonary disease　慢性閉塞性肺疾患（COPD）
admit　入院させる
ED　救急病棟（emergency department）

cancer　がん
caretaker　世話をする人

breathing　呼吸

Notes
(l. 2) stand over ~　～を見下ろすようにして立つ　　(l. 2) authoritative　高圧的な
(l. 5) sound like ~　～のように思われる　　(l. 6) why don't you ~?　～しませんか　　(l. 8) run away　逃げる
(l. 9) clarity　明確さ　　(l. 10) prior　前に　　(l. 11) relate　話す　　(l. 12) avert　そらす
(l. 12) mirror　そっくり模倣する　　(l. 13) tempo　調子　　(l. 13) rapport　信頼関係
(l. 14) turn one's attention to ~　～に注意を向ける　　(l. 16) tug on ~　～を強く引く　　(l. 17) in need　困っている
(l. 18) have a rough time　つらい思いをする　　(l. 19) scared　怯えた　　(l. 21) appointment　予約
(l. 22) not ~ anymore　もはや～ではない　　(l. 24) reassure　安心させる　　(l. 25) ensure　確実にする
(l. 25) provide an insight into ~　～を理解するうえでの手がかりとなる　　(l. 26) invaluable　非常に貴重な
(l. 26) tendency　傾向　　(l. 27) comfort　慰める

make any major movements during the night. *Gain the patient's trust by gaining that of his caregivers.*

Finally, I performed assessments, explaining each step along the way. *Engage patients in their own care.* As I showed him

5　how to use the pulse oximeter, I explained, "This helps us see how well you are breathing." Margaret interjected that his breathing trouble arose mainly at night ("We're always so worried when he goes to bed," she said). I assured her that we would watch his breathing through his monitor. *Remind them*

10　*that comfort is always nearby.* My time with Mr. Dixon showed me that my pediatric eyes—trained to see what my young patients couldn't, or wouldn't, tell me—would remain invaluable in this new field.

Before I left, Mr. Dixon told a few jokes. His daughter had

15　heard them a hundred times before—she rolled her eyes as he spoke. But at each punch line, we all laughed and laughed, like it was the first time.

| assessment　アセスメント，評価 |
| pulse oximeter　パルスオキシメーター，脈波型酸素飽和度計 |

Notes　(l. 4) engage　引き込む　　(l. 6) interject　不意に言う　　(l. 8) assure　保証する
(l. 15) roll one's eyes　（あきれて）目をくるりと回す　　(l. 16) punch line　（冗談の）おち

Reading Comprehension

次の英文が，本文の内容と一致する場合は T，一致しない場合は F を選びなさい。

1.（T / F）Beverly was an operating room nurse for 24 years before becoming a pediatric nurse.
2.（T / F）Mr. Dixon's wife died of cancer three years ago.
3.（T / F）Mr. Dixon tended to get out of bed without his cane.
4.（T / F）Beverly showed Margaret how to use the pulse oximeter.
5.（T / F）Mr. Dixon made the same jokes over and over.

音声を聴いて英文の空欄に適語を記入しなさい。また，完成した英文を日本語に直しなさい。

1. Who _____ _____ him while he was sick?

   _____

2. She _____ _____ a very nice person.

   _____

3. _____ _____ _____ try this one?

   _____

4. The horse jumped over the fence and _____ _____.

   _____

5. I _____ _____ _____ _____ last
   month.

   _____

日本文の意味に合うように，（ ）内の語句を並べかえて英文を作りなさい。

1. この情報は君にとって役に立つかもしれない。

   (you / to / be / use / this information / of / may).

   _____

2. 彼は再び道路へ注意を向けた。

   (again / attention / he / the road / turned / to / his).

   _____

3. まさかの時の友こそ真の友。(諺)

   (is / indeed / a friend / need / in / a friend).

   _____

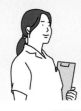

LEARN MORE

Nursing Terms and Expressions

次の日本文の空欄に入る語を下から選びなさい。

> かゆみ，下痢，充血，脱水症状，片頭痛，吐き気，麻痺，めまい

1. I have **congestion** in my nose from a cold.
   風邪で鼻の中が＿＿＿＿＿＿＿＿している。

2. Long distance runners often suffer from **dehydration**.
   長距離ランナーは，しばしば＿＿＿＿＿＿＿＿に苦しむ。

3. Some dairy products can cause **diarrhea**.
   乳製品のなかには，＿＿＿＿＿＿＿＿を引き起こすものもある。

4. His high fever caused **dizziness** and he fell.
   彼は高熱が原因で＿＿＿＿＿＿＿＿がして転倒した。

5. This ointment will reduce the **itching**.
   この軟膏で＿＿＿＿＿＿＿＿が和らぐでしょう。

6. He gets **migraines** once a week.
   彼は週に 1 回は＿＿＿＿＿＿＿＿になる。

7. She has a feeling of **nausea** from eating too much.
   彼女は食べ過ぎで＿＿＿＿＿＿＿＿がしている。

8. After the traffic accident, he suffered from **paralysis** of both his legs.
   交通事故の後，彼は両脚の＿＿＿＿＿＿＿＿に苦しんだ。

Column

　突然体調を崩した女性の様子を次のように描写する場面があります。"She could not catch her breath. She felt weak and dizzy." あるいは，次に診察する患者（スミス氏）の名前と症状について，看護師が医師に次のように伝えます。"Mr. Smith. Weak and dizzy all over."

　両方の場面に共通する weak and dizzy とは，医療機関などで患者の主訴（chief complaint）を表す典型的な表現です。身体に力が入らず（weak），めまいがする（dizzy）状態であることを患者が訴える場合に使われます。身体中がそのような状態なら weak and dizzy all over（略語で WADAO）となります。さらに痛みもあるなら weak and dizzy and hurt all over（略語で WADHAO）となります。

Unit 6
Bed Bath

The first day of the rest of my life.
* the rest of ~　～の残りの部分

Kathleen Hughes, MSN, RN, PNP-BC

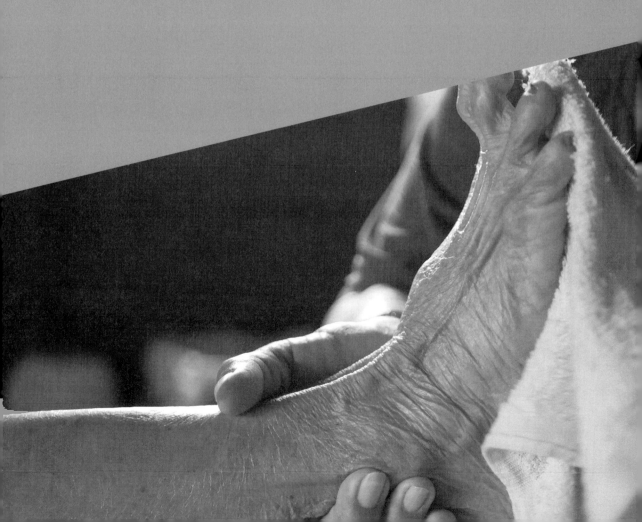

次の英語の意味に合う日本語を下から選びなさい。また，音声を聴いて発音しなさい。

1. basin _____   2. groin _____

3. bottom _____   4. exposure _____

5. dignity _____

尊厳，尻，洗面器，露出，股間

READING Essay 【Part 1】

CD 1-27 ▶ 27

エッセイの出だしを読んでみましょう。

Medical and Nursing Notes

cadaver	死体
dissection	解剖
bed bath	清拭
supply room	備品室
baby bottle	哺乳びん

Medical students start with cadaver dissection; nursing students start with bed baths. In preparation, I got the hair-washing cap from the supply room and warmed it in the microwave like a gas station burrito or a baby bottle. He wanted
5 the basin water as hot as he could stand it, but I worried that my version of hot water might be more extreme than his. I brought in at least six washcloths and towels. There were many deep, quiet breaths.

Notes (l. 2) in preparation 準備中で   (l. 2) hair-washing cap シャンプーキャップ   (l. 4) microwave 電子レンジ
(l. 4) gas station ガソリンスタンド   (l. 4) burrito （メキシコ料理の）ブリトー   (l. 5) stand 我慢する
(l. 6) extreme 極端な   (l. 6) bring in ~ ~を持ち込む   (l. 7) at least 少なくとも   (l. 7) washcloth 浴用タオル

Check the situation

Q1 看護学生のキャスリーン（筆者）が始めようとしていることは？

Q2 キャスリーンが心配していたことは？

Essay 【Part 2】 エッセイの続きを読んでみましょう。 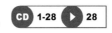 CD 1-28 ▶ 28

Medical and Nursing Notes

And then the only thing to do was to begin. I started with his upper body, his chest. He leaned forward for me to wash his back. I draped him with towels as his hospital johnny got a little damp. I washed his legs and feet, and made a mental note to see

drape	覆う
johnny	患者用ガウン

Notes (l. 1) and then （文頭で）それから   (l. 2) lean forward 前かがみになる   (l. 4) damp じめじめした
(l. 4) make a mental note to ~ 忘れないように~する

if there were any nail clippers in the supply room, not yet
having learned that nurses don't clip nails—whether because
it's a billable service, or curiously dangerous, or simply too time
consuming, I still don't know. He liked football, so I chatted
5 about the Colts and Notre Dame, careful not to insult his
Patriots or USC loyalty. His daughter was on another floor of
the hospital birthing his first grandchild, so he turned on the
newborn care channel. When he stood, not quite wobbly, to
wash his own groin, I held up his gown and watched out for his
10 IV and oxygen lines. Then I washed his bottom, donned him
in clean hospital wear, and sat him in the chair. Last, I used
the cap. As I massaged his scalp through it, and then dried and
combed his hair, he sighed like I was a master masseuse or a
magician who had cured his stubborn, inelastic lungs.

15 　　Should I describe his skin, his body, his face, so you can
see him as I did? It was pale but not translucent, aged but not
ancient, weathered but not beaten—and otherwise, I don't
remember. Though I believed I would never forget his name,
my first patient, it was gone from my mind within days, as if I'd
20 internalized HIPAA rules as a command to forget, to deidentify.
He had been a stranger to me when I arrived that morning,
and if I bumped into him on the street a week later, he'd be a
stranger again. In the moments of his exposure and my tending
to him, his skin was both everyone's and his alone, as my hands
25 were both mine and his.

　　Once he was clean and dry, I took another set of vitals,
made some notes, got my lunch, and left the hospital—that
intimidating and marvelous interior metropolis that I would

newborn care　新生児のケア

IV　点滴（intravenous）
oxygen line　酸素チューブ

scalp　頭皮

stubborn　（病気が）治りにくい
lung　肺

HIPAA　医療保険の相互運用性
と説明責任に関する法律（The
Health Insurance Portability and
Accountability Act）

tend to ~　～の世話をする

vitals　バイタルサイン（vital
signs）

Notes

(l. 1) nail clipper　爪切り　　　(l. 2) whether A or B　A であろうと B であろうと　　　(l. 3) billable　支払い請求可能な
(l. 3) curiously　（形容詞を修飾して）ひどく　　　(l. 3) time consuming　時間のかかる
(l. 5) Colts　インディアナポリスコルツ（アメリカンフットボール球団）
(l. 5) Notre Dame　ノートルダム（大学アメリカンフットボールチーム）　　　(l. 5) insult　侮辱する
(l. 6) Patriots　ニューイングランドペイトリオッツ（アメリカンフットボール球団）　　　(l. 6) USC　南カリフォルニア大学
(l. 6) loyalty　忠誠　　　(l. 8) not quite ~　すっかり～というわけではない　　　(l. 8) wobbly　足取りのおぼつかない
(l. 9) watch out for ~　～に注意する　　　(l. 10) don　服を着る　　　(l. 13) masseuse　マッサージ師
(l. 14) inelastic　弾力性のない　　　(l. 16) translucent　透き通るような　　　(l. 17) weathered　日に焼けた
(l. 17) beaten　疲れ果てた　　　(l. 17) ~ and otherwise　～やその他　　　(l. 19) as if ~　まるで～であるかのように
(l. 20) internalize　内在化する　　　(l. 20) deidentify　匿名化する　　　(l. 22) bump into ~　～にばったり出くわす
(l. 26) once ~　いったん～すると，～するとすぐに　　　(l. 28) intimidating　威嚇するような
(l. 28) marvelous　驚くべき　　　(l. 28) metropolis　大都市

like to call the Death Star for its massive, self-sufficient hive of wonder and industry, if not for the "death" part of the title. I have learned that the institution's preferred moniker, not entirely facetious, is Man's Greatest Hospital. Outside, it was

5　blindingly bright, a cerulean October sky, and the old stones paving Beacon Hill seemed wise.

　　An Ivy League degree and 15 years of teaching and writing did not prepare me any better than my mostly 20-something counterparts in the ways of giving a bed bath to a 72-year-

10　old man I'd never met. What might be different for me is that I have known many kinds of professional challenges. What might also be different is that I have lived enough longer to have attended my father's hospital-bound illness and death, and to have given birth to and cared for two young children. And

15　so when I washed this man, I was washing my father, I was washing my children; I became one of those people who cared for us. Though giving a bed bath is not anything like lecturing to AP students on Faulkner, or writing a newspaper article on gun control or university library funding or modern exorcisms,

20　I am not sure that either of those tasks made me hunker in a corner for five minutes, gathering myself before striding into the room. I've also never left a room feeling like I've had as simple and visceral an impact as I did that morning.

　　My work will get more technical and cerebral as I train

25　toward my master's degree and NP certification, and yet my work will remain what it was that first day: bearing witness to the body in wellness and suffering, and honoring the dignity in that body, the dignity in the desire for the most basic of human care.

Man's Greatest Hospital　ボストンにある Massachusetts General Hospital のあだ名

give a bed bath to ~　～を清拭する

attend　看護する
hospital-bound　病院に縛られた
give birth to ~　～を出産する
care for ~　～の世話をする

NP　ナースプラクティショナー（nurse practitioner）

Notes

(l. 1) Death Star　デススター（映画 *Star Wars* に登場する巨大な武装宇宙ステーション）
(l. 1) self-sufficient　独立した　　(l. 1) hive　人が忙しく働いている場所　　(l. 2) if not ~　～とは言わないが
(l. 3) moniker　あだ名　　(l. 3) not entirely ~　必ずしも～というわけではない　　(l. 4) facetious　おどけた
(l. 5) blindingly　目もくらむほど　　(l. 5) cerulean　空色の　　(l. 6) pave　舗装する
(l. 6) Beacon Hill　ビーコンヒル（ボストンの高級住宅地）　　(l. 7) Ivy League degree　アイヴィーリーグの学位
(l. 8) 20-something　（年齢が）20 代の　　(l. 9) counterpart　同等の相手
(l. 18) AP　アドバンストプレースメント（高校在学中に大学レベルの授業を受けて単位取得できるコース）
(l. 18) Faulkner　フォークナー（米国の小説家）　　(l. 19) funding　財政支援　　(l. 19) exorcism　悪魔払いの儀式
(l. 20) hunker　うずくまる　　(l. 21) gather oneself　心の準備をする　　(l. 21) stride　大股に歩く
(l. 23) visceral　本能的な，直感的な　　(l. 24) cerebral　知的な　　(l. 25) master's degree　修士号
(l. 25) certification　免許，認定　　(l. 25) and yet　それにもかかわらず　　(l. 26) bear witness to ~　～の証人となる

Reading Comprehension

次の英文が，本文の内容と一致する場合は T，一致しない場合は F を選びなさい。

1. (T / F) Kathleen chatted about the Colts and Notre Dame because the patient liked basketball.
2. (T / F) Kathleen's patient had a daughter, who was hospitalized in the same hospital because of her chest pain.
3. (T / F) Kathleen never forgot her first patient's name.
4. (T / F) Giving a bed bath to a 72-year-old patient was different from writing a newspaper article on gun control.
5. (T / F) Kathleen's work will become more professional and intellectual but it will remain what it was the first day.

EXERCISES   **Dictation & Translation**   CD 1-29 ▶ 29

音声を聴いて英文の空欄に適語を記入しなさい。また，完成した英文を日本語に直しなさい。

1. We'll eat _____ _____ _____ the cake tomorrow.

   _____

2. The thunderstorm lasted _____ _____ three hours.

   _____

3. Guess who I _____ _____ tonight?

   _____

4. Search and rescue teams were _____ _____ the survivors.

   _____

5. The changes will affect thousands, _____ _____ millions, of ordinary people.

   _____

EXERCISES   **Word Order & Translation**   CD 1-30 ▶ 30

日本文の意味に合うように，（ ）内の語句を並べかえて英文を作りなさい。

1. 君が勝とうが負けようが，僕は君のそばにいるよ。
   (by / win / your side / or / whether / I'll / you / be / lose).

   _____

2. 彼女が仕事を見つけるとすぐに，事態は好転した。
   (got / a job / better / she / once / things / found).

   _____

3. キャロルは昨日双子を出産した。
   (to / Carol / twins / birth / yesterday / gave).

   _____

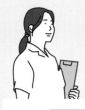

LEARN MORE

Nursing Terms and Expressions

次の日本文の空欄に入る語を下から選びなさい。

血圧，　呼吸数，　静脈，　徐脈，　体温，　動脈，　無呼吸，　頻脈，　不整脈，　脈拍数

---

1. **Arteries** are the blood vessels that deliver blood to the body. **Veins** are the blood vessels that return blood to the heart.

   ＿＿＿＿＿＿は，血液をからだに運ぶ血管である。＿＿＿＿＿＿は，血液を心臓へ戻す血管である。

2. Vital signs include **body temperature**, **pulse rate**, **respiration rate**, and **blood pressure**.

   バイタルサインには，＿＿＿＿＿＿，＿＿＿＿＿＿，＿＿＿＿＿＿，＿＿＿＿＿＿が含まれる。

3. **Bradycardia** is a very slow heart rate of less than 60 beats per minute. **Tachycardia** is a very fast heart rate of more than 100 beats per minute.

   ＿＿＿＿＿＿は，1分あたり60回未満の非常にゆっくりとした心拍数だ。＿＿＿＿＿＿は，1分あたり100回以上の非常に速い心拍数だ。

4. People with untreated sleep **apnea** stop breathing repeatedly during their sleep.

   睡眠時の＿＿＿＿＿＿を治療しないままの人は，睡眠中に繰り返し呼吸が止まる。

5. An **arrhythmia** is an irregular or abnormal heartbeat.

   ＿＿＿＿＿＿は，不規則なあるいは異常な心臓の鼓動だ。

Column

　brady- は「遅い」，tachy- は「急速な」という意味の連結形（combining form）です。また，-cardia は「心臓活動」という意味の連結形です。brady- + -cardia = bradycardia「遅い心臓活動」となり，tachy- + -cardia = tachycardia「急速な心臓活動」となります。

　apnea と arrhythmia に共通しているのは，「無…，非…」の意味を持つ接頭辞（prefix）の a-（r の前では ar-）です。a- + -pnea（「呼吸」の意味の連結形）= apnea となり，ar- + rhythm + -ia（「病気の状態」の意味の接尾辞）= arrhythmia となります。この a- は母音の前では an- となります。an- + -emia（「…な血液を有する状態」の意味の連結形）= anemia（貧血）や an- + -orexia（「食欲」の意味の連結形）= anorexia（食欲不振）があります。

　さて，米国の研修医の物語を読んでいる時に，患者の血管（静脈）が細くて採血に苦労する場面で aveinic という単語が出てきました。これはどのような成り立ちでできた語でしょうか？

Unit 7

A Nurse's Mother's Nurses

The RN, the CNA, the LPN ... she needed them all.

Donna Diers, PhD, RN, FAAN

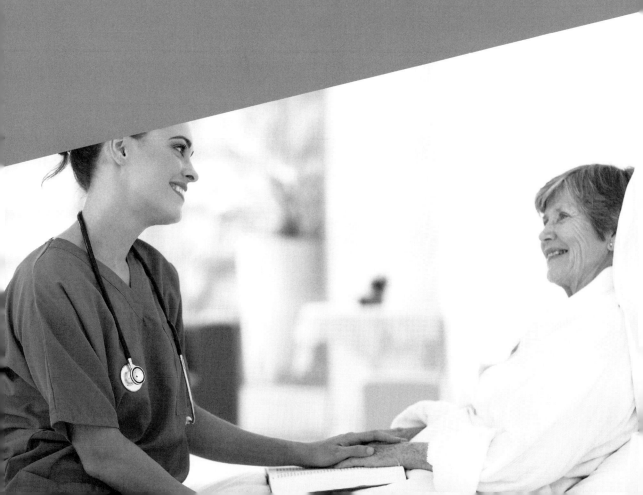

次の英語の意味に合う日本語を下から選びなさい。また，音声を聴いて発音しなさい。

1. cemetery   _____

2. osteoporosis   _____

3. arthritis   _____

4. commitment   _____

5. gratitude   _____

責任，関節炎，共同墓地，感謝，骨粗しょう症

READING   **Essay【Part 1】**   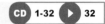 CD 1-32 ▶ 32

エッセイの出だしを読んでみましょう。

Medical and Nursing Notes

They walk toward me in the cemetery in a little town in Wyoming where we have just buried my mother: Linda, Carol, and Beverly, my mother's nurses.

Mom's osteoporosis had shrunk her from her proud 5'4" to
5 barely 5'. Arthritis had turned her hands into claws. Chronic obstructive pulmonary disease, which tethered her to an oxygen machine hidden discreetly behind a living room chair, had caused congestive heart failure. She was on enough medicines to fill the biggest plastic container the drug store carried.

10 I lived many guilty miles away in New England and my brother was a full day's drive south in Colorado. Dad took care of Mom and it had become a full-time job. The only time he really got away was just after dawn, while Mom was still asleep. He would meet an old friend for a quick round of golf on the
15 rough public course where the fairways were sagebrush and weeds and the greens were beige sand.

claw　かぎづめ
chronic obstructive pulmonary disease　慢性閉塞性肺疾患 (COPD)
oxygen machine　酸素濃縮器 (oxygen concentrator)

congestive heart failure　鬱血性心不全 (CHF)

Notes (l. 2) Wyoming　米国ワイオミング州　　(l. 2) bury　埋葬する　　(l. 4) shrink　縮ませる
(l. 4) 5'4"　5フィート4インチ（約162.5センチメートル）　　(l. 5) barely　やっと
(l. 5) 5'　5フィート（152.4センチメートル）　　(l. 6) tether　つなぐ　　(l. 7) discreetly　慎重に
(l. 10) guilty　気がとがめる，後ろめたい　　(l. 10) New England　ニューイングランド，米国北東部地方
(l. 11) Colorado　米国コロラド州　　(l. 13) dawn　夜明け　　(l. 15) fairway　（ゴルフコースの）フェアウェー
(l. 15) sagebrush　（雑草の）ヤマヨモギ　　(l. 16) weed　雑草
(l. 16) green　（ゴルフコースの）グリーン（putting green）　　(l. 16) beige　ベージュの

Check the situation

Q1 ドナ（筆者）の母親が罹っていた病気は何か，またその影響は？

Q2 妻の介護で忙しかったドナの父親が一息つけるのはいつ，その時何をして楽しんだか？

Mom and Dad decided they needed a little more help at home. I was relieved when I heard that community health nurses—my professional sisters—were going to be involved.

Carol came first. She was an LPN. Deeply tanned, she
5　looked as if she'd be more comfortable on a horse than in her Subaru and spoke only when she had something important to say. Carol took over the complicated medication regimen and the weekly "checkin' in."

Not long after, Linda joined the team. Linda was a nursing
10　assistant. The flaming red hair I remembered from when she was growing up a few years behind me had faded to dusky rose. Linda came two or three times a week to help Mom with her bath, a task that had Dad buffaloed. Mom and Linda clicked right away, and when I was there on one of my increasingly
15　frequent visits, Mom would rather have Linda help her. I would listen to them laugh as Linda jollied Mom through the shower that exhausted her. She was especially good with Mom's hair, about which she was deservedly vain. Hair care has always escaped me.

20　Mom began to slip a little bit more every time I flew in.

Without telling Mom and Dad, I went to the community health agency to see Beverly, an RN and case manager. I needed to sort out how to talk to my parents and shore them up. Bev, a calm, centered woman with huge brown eyes, suggested
25　that we all meet. When we did, and we sidled up to the question of palliative care, Mom refused to be dying.

Then one day Mom got breathless and Dad took her to the hospital. The X-ray showed lung cancer. When Mom told me about it on the phone as I was preparing to visit them, she

community health nurse　地域保健看護師，保健師

LPN　有資格実地看護師（licensed practical nurse），准看護師

medication regimen　投薬計画

nursing assistant　看護助手

community health agency　地域保健局
RN　登録看護師（registered nurse），正看護師
case manager　ケースマネージャー，ケアプラン担当者
centered　（精神的に）安定した

palliative care　緩和ケア

X-ray　X線写真
lung cancer　肺がん

Notes (l. 3) sister　女性の仲間　　(l. 4) tanned　日に焼けた　　(l. 5) as if ~　まるで~であるかのように
(l. 6) Subaru　（自動車ブランドの）スバル　　(l. 7) take over ~　~を引き継ぐ　　(l. 8) "checkin' in"　「訪問」
(l. 9) not long after　その後間もなく　　(l. 10) flaming　燃えるような　　(l. 11) grow up　成長する
(l. 11) dusky rose　くすんだバラ色の　　(l. 13) have A 過去分詞　A を~させる
(l. 13) buffalo　困らせる，まごつかせる　　(l. 13) click　意気投合する　　(l. 14) right away　すぐに
(l. 15) would rather ~　むしろ~したい　　(l. 15) have A 原形　A に~してもらう，A に~させる
(l. 16) jolly　おだてる　　(l. 17) be good with ~　~の扱いがうまい　　(l. 18) be vain about ~　~を自慢する
(l. 18) deservedly　当然　　(l. 19) escape　避ける　　(l. 20) slip　衰える　　(l. 20) every time ~　~するたびに
(l. 20) fly in　飛行機で着く　　(l. 23) sort out ~　~を解決する　　(l. 23) shore ~ up　~を支える
(l. 24) Bev　Beverly の愛称　　(l. 25) sidle up to ~　~におそるおそる近づく

seemed almost relieved. As a long-time smoker, she understood getting lung cancer. Although it probably wouldn't do much more than relieve her labored breathing, radiation was planned, in keeping with Mom's desire to be treated. Dad was tired and anxious about what might be next. We decided that short-term nursing home placement just up the street from their home would be best. Mom agreed.

I wanted her there too, in the hands of nurses—she already knew many of them, since her own mother had been a patient there, as had many of her friends. I helped with the move. Knowing I had a professional commitment in Arizona, I had packed my fancy dress. Mom loved clothes, so I modeled it for her in the nursing home. She liked it. She even said my hair looked good.

But Mom didn't settle in. She got twitchy and irritable. She began to call Dad at dawn, at noon. Dad started going to the nursing home early in the morning and spending most of the day with her. When I returned home from Arizona, the RN in the nursing home called and we had a conversation that led to a tricky dialogue with mom's physician about using morphine to make her more comfortable.

I got on a plane again.

Carol came to visit Mom in the nursing home. Dad was there. Mom was sleeping but woke to Carol's voice, smiled into the middle distance, took a deep breath, and died. I was somewhere over Iowa.

It took a small squad of all kinds of nurses to care for all of us.

Now, at the cemetery, I hug Linda, Carol, and Bev— a CNA, an LPN, and an RN—in wet, salty gratitude. They did for my mother what this fully credentialed, multiple degree-bearing nurse daughter couldn't do. They made all the difference to her—and to me.

---

labored breathing　苦しそうな呼吸，呼吸困難
radiation　放射線療法（radiation therapy）

nursing home　ナーシングホーム

physician　医師
morphine　（麻酔・鎮痛剤の）モルヒネ

care for ~　～の世話をする

CNA　認定看護助手（certified nursing assistant）

Notes
(l. 4) in keeping with ~　～を考慮して，～と一致して　　(l. 6) placement　（～へ）入れること
(l. 8) in the hands of ~　～の管理下に　　(l. 11) Arizona　米国アリゾナ州　　(l. 12) fancy dress　素敵な服
(l. 12) model　着て見せる　　(l. 15) settle in　落ち着く　　(l. 15) twitchy　そわそわした
(l. 19) lead to ~　～につながる　　(l. 20) tricky　微妙な　　(l. 24) smile into ~　～に微笑みかける
(l. 25) take a deep breath　深呼吸する　　(l. 26) Iowa　米国アイオワ州　　(l. 27) squad　チーム
(l. 30) credentialed　資格を持った　　(l. 31) degree-bearing　資格を持っている
(l. 31) make a difference　影響を与える

Reading Comprehension

次の英文が，本文の内容と一致する場合は T，一致しない場合は F を選びなさい。

1. (T / F) Carol was a registered nurse and in charge of the complicated medication regimen.

2. (T / F) Linda was a nursing assistant and soon got along with Donna's mother.

3. (T / F) Beverly was a case manager and suggested that Donna hold a family meeting.

4. (T / F) After Donna's mother was diagnosed with lung cancer, she moved to the long-term nursing home.

5. (T / F) When Donna's mother breathed her last breath, Carol was at her bedside.

EXERCISES　**Dictation & Translation**　　CD 1-34 ▶ 34

音声を聴いて英文の空欄に適語を記入しなさい。また，完成した英文を日本語に直しなさい。

1. His daughter will _____ _____ the business.

   _____

2. I want to become a nurse when I _____ _____.

   _____

3. Call me back _____ _____.

   _____

4. The roof leaks _____ _____ it rains.

   _____

5. The area is _____ _____ _____ _____ the rebels.

   _____

EXERCISES　**Word Order & Translation**　　CD 1-35 ▶ 35

日本文の意味に合うように，（　）内の語句を並べかえて英文を作りなさい。

1. 誰かにそのレポートのコピーを君に送らせよう。

   (someone / you / the report / of / I'll / send / a copy / have).

   _____

2. 彼の行動は言葉と一致していなかった。

   (his words / with / not / his actions / keeping / in / were).

   _____

3. その研究がその新薬の開発につながった。

   (to / the new drug / led / of / the research / the development).

   _____

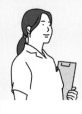

Nursing Terms and Expressions

米国の看護師について，次の表の（　）内に入る語を下から選びなさい。

English	definition	Japanese
charge nurse	a nurse who is in charge of one section of a hospital	主任看護師
1.(　　　　　　　　) **nurse**	a nurse who has a degree in nursing and who has passed an exam to be allowed to work in a particular state	正看護師
2.(　　　　　　　　) **nurse**	a nurse member of the surgical team, responsible for activities of the operating room outside the sterile field	外回り看護師
flight nurse	a registered nurse who accompanies seriously ill patients during air 5.(　　　　　　　)	フライトナース
head nurse (= nurse manager)	a nurse with overall 6.(　　　　　　) for the supervision of the administrative and clinical aspects of nursing care	看護師長
3.(　　　　　　) **practical nurse**	a nurse who has passed an exam to be allowed to work under the direction of a registered nurse or a doctor	准看護師
nurse-midwife	a professional nurse who specializes in the care of women throughout 7.(　　　　　　　), delivery, and the postpartum period	看護助産師
nurse practitioner	a nurse who is trained to do some of the work that is usually done by a 8.(　　　　　　)	ナースプラクティショナー
public health nurse (= community health nurse)	a nurse employed by a hospital or social-service agency to perform public health services and especially to visit and provide care for sick persons in a 9.(　　　　　　　)	保健師
4.(　　　　　　) **nurse**	a nurse who directly assists the surgeon in an operating room	器械出し看護師

circulating, **licensed**, **registered**, **scrub**	community, doctor, pregnancy, responsibility, transport

Column

　日本の准看護師に相当する licensed practical nurse（LPN）がさらに高い専門的知識や能力を身につけて，日本の正看護師に相当する registered nurse（RN）になるためのプログラムを紹介する広告には，次のように書かれています。

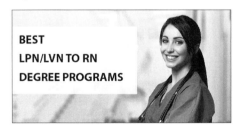

BEST
LPN/LVN TO RN
DEGREE PROGRAMS

　LPN/LVN の LVN は licensed vocational nurse の頭文字です。米国ではカリフォルニア州とテキサス州だけは，licensed practical nurse ではなく licensed vocational nurse という名称が使われています。

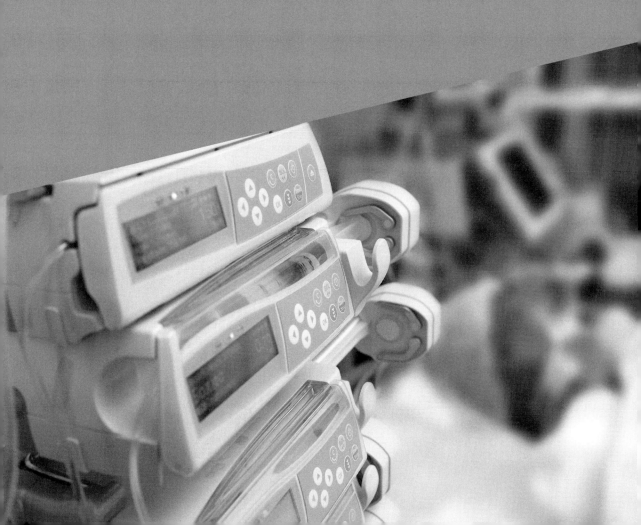

Unit 8
A Place for Palliative Care

Families have a right to know the true meaning of 'survival.'

Carrie A. Bennett, MS, CNS-BC

次の英語の意味に合う日本語を下から選びなさい。また，音声を聴いて発音しなさい。

1. terminology _____   **2.** chemotherapy _____

3. leukemia _____   **4.** antibiotic _____

5. kidney _____

抗生物質，化学療法，腎臓，用語，白血病

READING   **Essay 【Part 1】**   CD 1-37 ▶ 37

エッセイの出だしを読んでみましょう。

Medical and Nursing Notes

I haven't seen her yet, but my husband has been updating me on her condition. He doesn't understand medical terminology, and his updates have lost some detail in translation, but I'm able to piece together a story that sounds logical: my

5 mother-in-law's condition is grave. The chemotherapies used to put her leukemia into remission have savaged her body, and she doesn't have the reserve to fight this new respiratory infection. I don't know how to tell him this, so I just hold him and say that we should go and be with her. I'm a nurse, but I'm also his wife.

10 When I do see her, she looks just as I'd envisioned. She is sedated and intubated. The monitor above her bed shows a blood pressure of 68/46, a heart rate of 174. I expect to hear a critical alarm, but the monitor has been silenced. Her face is flushed, and her extremities are cool. She is on vasopressors

15 and antiarrhythmics. She is on antibiotics, antifungals, and antivirals. A continuous renal replacement therapy machine sits beside her bed, waiting to dialyze her, but her pressures are too low. She is third spacing. I subtly pull the white sheet up to hide the fluid weeping from her extremities—something her children

20 don't need to see.

remission 寛解（完治ではないが病状がおさまっておだやかな状態）
respiratory infection 呼吸器感染症

sedate 鎮静剤で落ち着かせる
intubate （気管などに）挿管する
blood pressure 血圧
heart rate 心拍数
critical alarm 危篤であることを知らせる警報音
extremity （複数形で）両手両足
vasopressor 昇圧薬
antiarrhythmic 抗不整脈薬
antifungal 抗真菌薬
antiviral 抗ウイルス薬
renal replacement therapy 腎機能代替療法
dialyze 透析する
third space 血漿成分が細胞内でも血管内でもない場所（third space）に溜まる
fluid 分泌液

Notes (l. 3) translation　言い換え　　(l. 4) piece together ~　～をつなぎ合わせて理解する　　(l. 5) mother-in-law　義母
(l. 5) grave　深刻な　　(l. 6) savage　激しく攻撃する　　(l. 7) reserve　余力　　(l. 10) envision　予想する
(l. 14) flushed　赤くなって　　(l. 18) subtly　巧妙に　　(l. 19) weep　しみ出る

Check the situation

Q1 キャリー（筆者）の義母が罹っていた病気は？　いま罹っている病気は？

Q2 キャリーの義母が服用している薬は？　受けている治療法は？

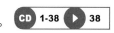

Medical and Nursing Notes

physician 医師

Physicians say she has a chance of surviving with continued aggressive treatment. She is a "full code." Family gathers around her, holding onto the chance, misinterpreting survival as recovery. I don't know how to tell them the difference, so I
5 stand aside. I'm a nurse, but I'm also their in-law.

A family meeting is called and I'm invited to attend. Physicians tell the family that her lungs are damaged, her liver is damaged, her kidneys are damaged, and her heart is damaged. They don't know how her brain is doing, but think it
10 may be damaged as well. They reiterate the chance of survival and answer the one question I'd posed to them earlier: would a palliative care consultation be appropriate at this point? "No," they tell us, "she can still survive." Her family agrees to pursue aggressive care. She would want to survive, they reason. But
15 survival continues to be mistaken for recovery, and no health care provider has explained otherwise. The physicians excuse themselves to insert a line in her femoral artery. I sit with the family. I'm their in-law, but I'm also a nurse.

I'm a nurse with years of experience in palliative care.
20 Years of encountering similar situations: families caught up in a reality created by a misunderstanding of the medical world and its language. I carefully open up discussion and hold the palliative care consultation the family so desperately needs. We talk about the implications of her damaged organ systems—
25 chronic ventilator support, dialysis, artificial nutrition— the likelihood of brain damage. We talk about her definition of quality of life—traveling the country with her beloved husband, hosting grand holiday gatherings, and reading to her dear, sweet grandbabies. And in our discussion it becomes

aggressive 積極的な
treatment 治療
"full code" 「フルコード」心拍停止状態で心肺蘇生術を受ける状態

lung 肺

liver 肝臓
heart 心臓
brain 脳

palliative care 緩和ケア

health care provider 保健医療提供者

femoral artery 大腿動脈

organ system 器官系，臓器系

chronic 長期にわたる
ventilator 人工呼吸器
dialysis 透析
artificial nutrition 人工的栄養補給法
brain damage 脳損傷
quality of life 生活の質（QOL）

Notes (l. 3) hold onto ~ ～にすがる，～にしがみつく　　(l. 3) misinterpret A as B　A を B と誤解する
(l. 5) stand aside　傍観する　　(l. 5) in-law　姻戚（結婚によって親類関係となった者）　　(l. 10) ~ as well　～もまた
(l. 10) reiterate　繰り返し言う　　(l. 11) pose　提起する　　(l. 12) consultation　相談
(l. 12) appropriate　ふさわしい　　(l. 13) pursue　追い求める　　(l. 14) reason　判断する
(l. 15) mistake A for B　A を B と間違える　　(l. 16) otherwise　違うふうに
(l. 16) excuse oneself　詫びる，弁解する　　(l. 17) insert　挿入する　　(l. 20) encounter　直面する
(l. 20) (be) caught up in ~　～に巻き込まれる，～で動けなくなる　　(l. 22) open up ~　～を開始する
(l. 23) desperately　すごく　　(l. 24) implication　（複数形で）予想される結果，影響　　(l. 26) likelihood　可能性
(l. 26) definition　（範囲などの）限定　　(l. 27) beloved　最愛の　　(l. 28) grand　大がかりな

apparent that she wouldn't be satisfied with simply surviving. She would want to recover—an unlikely feat at this point in her illness.

5　The physicians are updated and her code status is changed. Family gathers around her bedside and she dies a short while later. They're sad but appear at peace with their decision to let her die with dignity. The physicians gather around her bedside too, offering condolences. Their demeanor is professional, but they appear defeated—an ICU patient they couldn't save. I'm

10　sad for all of them, including the physicians.

The finality of death is a concept so difficult to grasp. And, somehow, the medical culture has come to equate the finality of death with the ultimate failure—a detrimental view that precludes acceptance of palliative care services into most

15　intensive care settings. My mother-in-law's death was not a failure, but rather an outcome of our attempt to respect her wish to *live*, not merely survive. Failure would have been to keep her alive, chronically dependent on a ventilator and dialysis and fed through a tube.

code status　コードステータス（心拍停止状態の場合にどのような対応をするかという取り決め）

die with dignity　尊厳をもって死ぬ

ICU　集中治療室（intensive care unit）

Notes　(l. 1) be satisfied with ~　～に満足している　　(l. 2) unlikely　起こりそうもない　　(l. 2) feat　芸当，離れ業
(l. 6) at peace　安心して　　(l. 8) condolence　（複数形で）哀悼の言葉　　(l. 8) demeanor　態度
(l. 9) defeated　（戦いに）敗れた　　(l. 11) finality　結末　　(l. 12) somehow　どういうわけか
(l. 12) equate A with B　A を B と同一視する　　(l. 13) ultimate　究極の　　(l. 13) detrimental　有害な
(l. 14) preclude　あらかじめ排除する　　(l. 18) dependent　頼っている　　(l. 18) feed　食べ物を食べさせる

Reading Comprehension

次の英文が，本文の内容と一致する場合は T，一致しない場合は F を選びなさい。

1. (T / F) When doctors said that Carrie's mother-in-law had a chance of survival, the family didn't understand the difference between survival and recovery.

2. (T / F) Carrie's mother-in-law's lungs, liver, kidneys and stomach were damaged.

3. (T / F) Carrie was an experienced nurse, but she had little experience in palliative care.

4. (T / F) The family discussed the mother's quality of life.

5. (T / F) The mother-in-law's death was an outcome of our attempt to respect her wish to survive.

音声を聴いて英文の空欄に適語を記入しなさい。また，完成した英文を日本語に直しなさい。

1. They were finally able to _____ _____ the whole story of her death.

   _____

2. The child _____ _____ her mother.

   _____

3. They advertised the new car on television, and in newspapers _____ _____.

   _____

4. They were _____ _____ _____ the riots.

   _____

5. She never felt really _____ _____ with herself.

   _____

日本文の意味に合うように，（　）内の語句を並べかえて英文を作りなさい。

1. 彼はしばしば電話で私を私の母親と間違える。
   (my mother / often / for / the phone / mistakes / he / on / me).

   _____

2. 私はあなたがやったその仕事に本当に満足している。
   (did / the job / satisfied / am / you / with / really / I).

   _____

3. 金と幸福を同一視するのは間違いだ。
   (money / to / is / happiness / equate / it / with / a mistake).

   _____

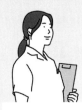

Nursing Terms and Expressions

次の日本文の空欄に入る語を下から選びなさい。

坐薬, 市販薬, 抗生物質, 緩下薬（かんげ）, 去痰薬（きょたん）, 充血除去薬, 制酸薬, 鎮静薬

---

1. Pregnant women should use **antacids** cautiously during pregnancy.
   妊娠した女性は，妊娠中は注意して＿＿＿＿＿＿＿＿を使わなければならない。

2. **Antibiotics** are medicines used to prevent and treat bacterial infections.
   ＿＿＿＿＿＿＿＿は，細菌感染症を防いだり治療したりするのに使われる薬だ。

3. Most **decongestants** should only be used between 1 and 4 times a day.
   ほとんどの＿＿＿＿＿＿＿は，1日につき1回から4回のみ使用されなければならない。

4. Wet coughs are sometimes treated with **expectorants**.
   湿性咳は＿＿＿＿＿＿＿で治療されることもある。

5. **Laxatives** can help relieve and prevent constipation.
   ＿＿＿＿＿＿＿は，便秘を和らげて治療するのに役立つことができる。

6. Doctors prescribe **sedatives** to treat conditions like anxiety and sleep disorders.
   医師は，不安や睡眠障害のような状態を治療するために＿＿＿＿＿＿＿を処方する。

7. **Suppositories** are solid medications that enter the body through the rectum, vagina, or urethra.
   ＿＿＿＿＿＿＿は，直腸，膣，尿道を通じてからだに入る固形薬だ。

8. **OTC drugs** aren't as strong as prescription drugs.
   ＿＿＿＿＿＿＿は処方薬ほど強力でない。

Column

　大ヒットした米国の医療ドラマ *ER*（『ER 緊急救命室』）には，負傷者多数の triage（負傷者選別）で大混乱の ER (emergency room) にやってきた精神科の常連患者に対して，医師が Vitamin H を処方するよう指示を出す場面があります。Vitamin H とは antipsychotic（抗精神病薬）の Haldol のことで，Vitamin と薬品名の頭文字 H を組み合わせて，その薬を栄養素のビタミンのように呼ぶ表現です。他にも，diuretic の Lasix を指す Vitamin L，anti-inflammatory（抗炎症薬）の Motrin を指す Vitamin M，narcotic antagonist（麻薬拮抗薬）の Narcan を指す Vitamin N，antidepressant の Prozac を指す Vitamin P，anesthetic の Versed を指す Vitamin V などがあります。diuretic, antidepressant, anesthetic とは，それぞれどんな薬でしょうか？

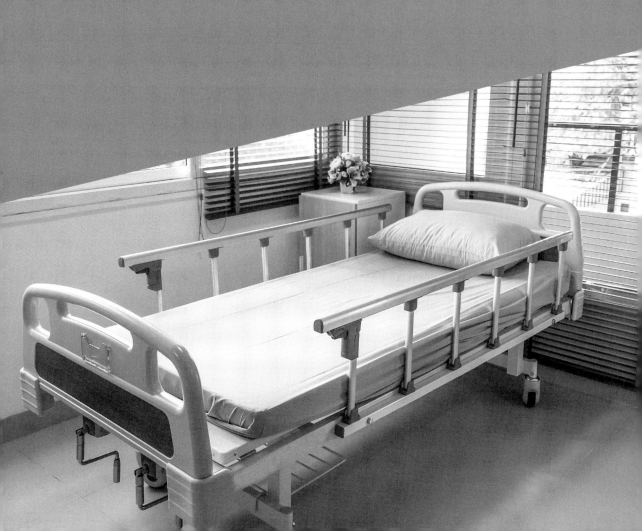

Unit 9

My Turn

A retired physician recalls how a nurse helped him out of a predicament as a new intern.

* predicament　窮地

Michael M. Bloomfield, MD

次の英語の意味に合う日本語を下から選びなさい。また，音声を聴いて発音しなさい。

1. reputation　_____　**2.** differential　_____

3. respiration　_____　**4.** compassion　_____

5. condolence　_____

思いやり，分類，哀悼，評判，呼吸

READING　**Essay 〔Part 1〕**　CD 2-02 ▶ 42

エッセイの出だしを読んでみましょう。

Medical and Nursing Notes

　　Medicine was my first rotation as an intern. At University Hospitals of Cleveland, the medicine rotation had a particularly intimidating reputation and a red-hot I was not. I was terrified.

　　On morning rounds every day our entourage of physicians,
5　nurses, and students would go room to room discussing each patient. I can still see the open door to Mrs. Finkelstein's room near the morning sunlight at the end of the hallway. Mrs. Finkelstein was old and was dying. And every morning when we walked in, her husband was sitting there next to the bed,
10　holding her hand. He told us regularly how many years they had been together. We each dreaded being the one on call when she died.

intern　インターン，1年目の研修医（resident）
medicine　内科

round　回診
physician　医師

on call　待機して，当直の

Notes　(l. 2) Cleveland　クリーブランド（米国オハイオ州の工業都市）
(l. 3) intimidating　人を怖がらせるような　　(l. 3) red-hot　熱烈な人　　(l. 3) terrified　怯えた
(l. 4) entourage　側近，取り巻き　　(l. 7) at the end of ~　～の突き当りの　　(l. 7) hallway　廊下
(l. 9) next to ~　～の隣の　　(l. 11) dread　ひどく恐れる

Check the situation
Q1　マイケル（筆者）がクリーブランドの大学病院で経験したのは何か？
Q2　フィンケルスタインの病状は？

Medical and Nursing Notes

Call was every third night and was grueling. One night when it was my turn, my senior resident pulled me aside after sign-out rounds and said that Mrs. Finkelstein would probably die on my shift. I wasn't ready. In medical school they taught us
5 everything about keeping someone alive, but no one ever told me what to do when a patient dies. I had never pronounced a patient dead before. No one had even explained to me how to tell if someone is dead.

He could tell. He said take your time. Be respectful. Be
10 methodical. Be confident. Appreciate the meaning of the moment for the family. Listen to the heart, look for respiratory effort. Talk straight. Stay for as long as the family needs you. And then he left me in charge of the floor for the night.

Call was mayhem. Always. The night was spent frantically
15 admitting patients, taking histories, doing physical exams, checking labs, writing orders, starting ivs, talking to family members, flaming broth tubes for blood cultures, doing manual white cell differentials, and the 10,000 other things that an intern had to do in those days on a medicine rotation at
20 University Hospitals of Cleveland preparing for the assault at morning rounds. Sleep was never really an option.

Somewhere in the middle of the night and the chaos a nurse came up to me with that look, and I knew. I wasn't ready. She could tell. She came with me.

25 He was there, holding her hand as always, eyes wide. His whole world depended on me. I walked in quietly, looked for respiration and listened to her heart for a long time. Nothing. I took the stethoscope out of my ears and looked at him with genuine compassion and said, "I'm so sorry." He looked down

Medical and Nursing Notes (margin glossary):

call 夜勤

resident 研修医（senior resident は「後期研修医」の意味があるが ここでは「先輩の研修医」の意味）

pronounce ~ dead ～の死亡を宣告する

heart 心臓
respiratory 呼吸のための

in charge of ~ ～を担当して

admit 入院させる
history 病歴
physical exam 身体検査（physical examination）
lab 臨床検査（laboratory test）
iv 静脈点滴（intravenous）
flame （殺菌のために）火に当てる
broth tube 培養液の入った試験管
blood culture 血液培養
white cell 白血球（white blood cell）

stethoscope 聴診器

Notes
(l. 1) every ~ ～ごとに (l. 1) grueling へとへとに疲れさせる (l. 2) pull ~ aside ～を脇へ連れ出す
(l. 3) sign-out 退出時の (l. 9) take one's time 急がず慎重にやる (l. 9) respectful 敬意を表する
(l. 10) methodical 几帳面な (l. 10) confident 自信をもった (l. 10) appreciate 正しく認識する
(l. 11) look for ~ ～をさがす (l. 12) as long as ~ ～する間は (l. 14) mayhem 大混乱
(l. 14) spend 時間 ~ing ～することに時間を費やす (l. 14) frantically 大慌てで
(l. 20) assault 言葉による激しい攻撃，非難 (l. 22) in the middle of ~ ～の中ごろに (l. 22) chaos 大混乱
(l. 23) come up to ~ ～に近寄る (l. 26) depend on ~ ～しだいである (l. 29) genuine 心からの

at the bed, dazed, and we stood there in silence, sharing the weight of the moment.

That's when it happened. Mrs. Finkelstein breathed an enormous sigh! We all froze. I was mortified. Mr. Finkelstein
5 looked at her—looked at me—looked at her—looked at me.

"What was that?!" he said. I tried to look calm. "Well, is she dead or isn't she?" he yelled. Inside, I was reeling. *What the hell? Is she dead or isn't she? Four years of medical school and I can't tell if someone's dead?!* Time froze—the moment remains
10 suspended in my memory still. I don't know how long we stood there, but it felt like such a long time.

"After a person dies there are last gasps," the nurse explained to him quietly as if it came from both of us. "Not unusual." I nodded authoritative agreement, expressed my
15 deepest condolences, stayed as long as I possibly could, and went back to the 10,000 things. And I have remained indebted to that nameless nurse of the night ever since. And to so many others throughout my career who quietly saved me.

last gasp　最後の喘ぎ

(l. 1) dazed　茫然として　　(l. 1) in silence　無言で　　(l. 4) be mortified　当惑している　　(l. 7) reel　動揺する
(l. 7) What the hell?　なんだって？　　(l. 10) suspended　停止した　　(l. 11) feel like ~　~のような感じがする
(l. 13) as if ~　まるで~であるかのように　　(l. 14) authoritative　権威のある　　(l. 14) agreement　同意
(l. 16) indebted to ~　~に恩を受けている　　(l. 17) ever since　それ以来ずっと　　(l. 17) so many ~　非常に多くの~

Reading Comprehension

次の英文が，本文の内容と一致する場合は T，一致しない場合は F を選びなさい。

1. (T / F) Medical students learn not only what to do to keep patients alive but also what to do when patients die.

2. (T / F) The senior resident left the floor without a word.

3. (T / F) After interns spent the on-call night doing many things, they were under assault from doctors at morning rounds.

4. (T / F) When Mrs. Finkelstein gasped her last, Michael was calm and knew what to do.

5. (T / F) Michael has been indebted to the nurse who explained the last gasp to Mr. Finkelstein.

音声を聴いて英文の空欄に適語を記入しなさい。また，完成した英文を日本語に直しなさい。

1. _____ _____ _____. We still have lots of time.

   _____

2. How long have you been _____ _____ a job?

   _____

3. Who is _____ _____ _____ the ICU?

   _____

4. The family sat eating _____ _____.

   _____

5. I got my first job in 1985 and I've been working _____ _____.

   _____

日本文の意味に合うように，（　）内の語句を並べかえて英文を作りなさい。

1. 彼女は映画の最中に眠り込んだ。

   (the movie / the middle / asleep / she / of / in / fell).

   _____

2. 個々の治療計画はがんのタイプ次第だ。

   (the type / on / treatment plans / cancer / individual / of / depend).

   _____

3. ジョンはまるで彼女に以前一度も会ったことがないかのようにふるまった。

   (before / acted / seen / had / as / John / her / never / he / if).

   _____

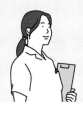

LEARN MORE

Nursing Terms and Expressions

臓器について，次の表の（　）内に入る語を下から選びなさい。また，イラストからその臓器を指す記号を選びなさい。

English	definition	Japanese	イラスト
bladder	an organ inside the body that stores 5.(　　　　　) until it can be excreted	膀胱	15.(　)
esophagus	the tube in the body that carries food from the 6.(　　　　　) to the stomach	食道	16.(　)
heart	the organ in the chest that sends the 7.(　　　　) around your body	11.(　　)	17.(　)
small 1.(　　　　)	the tube in your body that food goes into after it has passed through your stomach	12.(　　)	18.(　)
2.(　　　　)	either of a pair of small organs in the body that remove waste matter from the blood and produce urine	腎臓	19.(　)
3.(　　　　)	a large organ in the body that cleans the blood and produces bile	肝臓	20.(　)
4.(　　　　)	either of the two breathing organs in the chest that supply 8.(　　　　　) to the blood	肺	21.(　)
pancreas	an organ in the body that produces 9.(　　　　) and a liquid that helps the body to digest food	膵臓	22.(　)
spleen	an organ near the stomach that controls the quality of your blood	13.(　　)	23.(　)
stomach	an organ in the body where 10.(　　　　) is digested	14.(　　)	24.(　)

liver, lung, intestine, kidney	blood, food, insulin, mouth, oxygen, urine	胃，小腸，心臓，脾臓

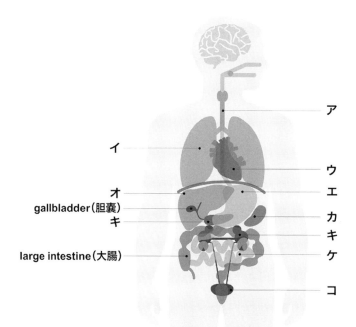

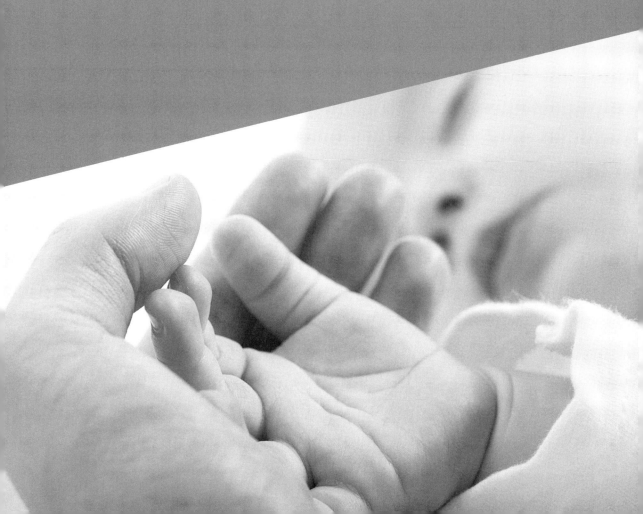

Unit 10
Big Love

How "the baby" became "my son."

Marcia Gardner, MA, RN, CPNP, CPN

次の英語の意味に合う日本語を下から選びなさい。また，音声を聴いて発音しなさい。

1. meconium _____ 　　　**2.** intervention _____

3. incision _____ 　　　**4.** pneumothorax _____

5. literature _____

文献，切開，胎便，気胸，介入

READING　　**Essay【Part 1】**　　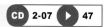

エッセイの出だしを読んでみましょう。

Medical and Nursing Notes

　　　We named our first child Robbie, after my father, who died when I was in high school. I was 31 years old when Robbie was born. Although my pregnancy was completely normal, I never went into labor. By the time the obstetrician decided to induce

5　labor, I was more than 42 weeks into my pregnancy.

　　　We'd planned on a typical, long, epidural-supported first labor, but a good situation quickly turned bad. Late decelerations, decreased variability, decreased movement, and meconium in the amniotic fluid—they all happened so fast

10　that I barely had time to grasp the need for all the associated interventions. In the end, I underwent an emergency C-section.

pregnancy　妊娠
labor　陣痛，分娩
obstetrician　産科医
induce　（陣痛を）誘発する
epidural-supported　硬膜外麻酔
（epidural anesthesia）に支えられた
late deceleration　遅発一過性徐脈
decreased variability　基線細変動
減少 （decreased baseline
variability）
decreased movement　胎動減少
（decreased fetal movement）
amniotic fluid　羊水
undergo　（手術・治療などを）受
ける
emergency C-section　緊急帝王切
開

Notes　(l. 1) name A after B　B にちなんで A と命名する　　(l. 4) by the time ~　～する時までには
(l. 5) more than ~　～以上　　(l. 6) plan on ~　～するつもりである　　(l. 9) so ~ that ...　非常に～なので…
(l. 10) barely　ほとんど～ない　　(l. 10) grasp　把握する，理解する　　(l. 11) in the end　結局

Check the situation

　Q1　マーシャ（筆者）が妊娠期間に困ったことは？

　Q2　マーシャの分娩中，最終的に取った手段は？

Medical and Nursing Notes

When I awoke in the recovery room, with my abdominal incision burning, I learned Robbie weighed slightly more than 5 lbs. Three weeks earlier, his estimated weight had been more than 8 lbs. Meetings with neonatologists began. Conversations
5　were laden with laboratory data. "The baby," as they called him, had a decreased white cell count. A serious infection. Thrombocytopenia. Pneumothorax. "The baby" needed head ultrasonography and could have developmental problems in the future.

10　I was bombarded with so much information, such a multitude of potential problems, and was spending so little time with my newborn son that after two days he was beginning to sound like nothing more than a complex set of medical conditions.

15　My loved ones could offer me no reprieve. My husband, focused on the joy of a newborn son, didn't grasp the potential long-term implications of Robbie's problems. My mother searched for reasons for his condition, concluding that it was my fault for working too hard and having pets in the house while
20　pregnant. Conversations with my siblings can be summed up as: "My friend had a baby who was little and that baby turned out great."

It was Robbie's nurses who helped me see beyond his medical challenges. They congratulated me on the birth of
25　a sweet and beautiful baby boy, which no one else had done. They hurried into my room as his physicians hurried out saying "we don't know yet." They stayed with me as I cried. The nurses called him Robbie, not "the baby." They pointed out my son's miniature hands and complimented me on his

recovery room　回復室	
abdominal　腹部の	
burn　焼けるように痛む	
neonatologist　新生児専門医	
laboratory data　検査値	
white cell count　白血球（white blood cell）数	
infection　感染症	
thrombocytopenia　血小板減少（症）	
ultrasonography　超音波検査法	
developmental　発育上の	

pregnant　妊娠した

physician　医師

Notes

(l. 3) lb.　ポンド（pound）．0.454 キログラム．5 ポンドは約 2.3 キログラム．8 ポンドは約 3.6 キログラム
(l. 3) estimated　見積もりの，推定の　　(l. 5) be laden with ~　~をたくさん含んだ　　(l. 8) in the future　今後は
(l. 10) bombard　攻め立てる　　(l. 10) a multitude of ~　たくさんの~　　(l. 13) sound like ~　~のように聞こえる
(l. 13) nothing more than ~　ただ~にすぎない　　(l. 15) loved ones　家族　　(l. 15) reprieve　一時的軽減
(l. 17) implication　（複数形で）影響，結果　　(l. 18) search for ~　~を探し求める　　(l. 20) sibling　きょうだい
(l. 20) sum up　要約する　　(l. 21) turn out ~　結局~となる　　(l. 23) It is A who ~　~なのは A である
(l. 23) see beyond ~　~の先を見通す　　(l. 24) congratulate A on B　A を B のことで祝う
(l. 27) stay with ~　~に付き添う　　(l. 28) point out ~　~を指し示す　　(l. 29) miniature　普通よりずっと小さい

long fingers. They admired his huge, clear blue eyes, his soft baby hair, and his big gummy smile. They reassured me that there was a lot that was baby-like, not diseaselike, about him.

5　After five days I was discharged, and Robbie was moved to the transitional nursery. The medical staff continued to test his blood and give him ultrasonography, X-rays, and hip evaluations. I visited every day, hearing results of each and every new test given to "the baby" as I sat by my son's bassinet.

Rita, the nurse in the transitional nursery, never left my
10　side when I needed her, always making time to listen to my worries. When I came to visit, she told me Robbie was "such a cute little guy" and had "such a big personality." She picked him up and slung him over her shoulder, showing me that he was strong. She held him upright and spoke straight to his face.
15　"You fresh little guy," she scolded, her voice warm and teasing. "You're giving your mom a lot of grief."

Just out of school, I'd worked in a level III neonatal intensive care unit. At 22 years old, I made a point of finding beautiful features in every tiny newborn face and of showing
20　mothers that their babies, although vulnerable, were also strong and could be handled, held, and hugged. But I'd done so because that's what the literature and my teachers had instructed me to do. It was only when I became a mother that I truly understood the power of our words and deeds.

25　Nine days after Robbie was born, as I finally headed home with my son, I looked back at Rita. She nodded, smiling, as though she knew that we were ready to take this step and that we would thrive. And we did. Robbie is 15 years old now and he plays the piano beautifully (those nurses were right about
30　his fingers), including a particularly memorable version of Fleetwood Mac's "Big Love."

diseaselike	病気のような
discharge	退院させる
transitional nursery	移行期の育児室
X-ray	X線
hip	股関節
bassinet	新生児用かご型ベッド
neonatal intensive care unit	新生児集中治療室（NICU）

Notes
(l. 1) admire　称賛する　　(l. 2) gummy smile　歯ぐきを見せた微笑み　　(l. 2) reassure　安心させる
(l. 10) make time to ~　~するための時間を作る　　(l. 13) sling　（無造作に）ほうる　　(l. 14) upright　まっすぐに
(l. 15) scold　叱る　　(l. 15) teasing　からかうような　　(l. 16) grief　深い悲しみ
(l. 18) make a point of ~ing　必ず~するよう努力する　　(l. 20) vulnerable　傷つきやすい，脆弱な
(l. 23) It is only when ~ that ...　~して初めて…だ　　(l. 26) as though ~　まるで~であるかのように
(l. 27) be ready to ~　喜んで~する　　(l. 28) thrive　栄える，成功する
(l. 31) Fleetwood Mac　イングランド出身のロックバンド（"Big Love" は 1987 発表のシングル）

Reading Comprehension

次の英文が，本文の内容と一致する場合は T，一致しない場合は F を選びなさい。

1. (T / F) Robbie was named after his father.
2. (T / F) Conversations with neonatologists were full of laboratory data.
3. (T / F) It was Marcia's fault that her baby was born with medical problems.
4. (T / F) Rita was the only nurse that helped Marcia see beyond her son's medical challenges.
5. (T / F) When Marcia worked in the NICU, she made it a point to find a beautiful feature in every newborn face.

EXERCISES　**Dictation & Translation**　　CD 2-09 ▶ 49

音声を聴いて英文の空欄に適語を記入しなさい。また，完成した英文を日本語に直しなさい。

1. _____ _____ _____, we decided to go to Australia.

   _____

2. Who knows what will happen _____ _____ _____?

   _____

3. This is _____ _____ _____ a rumor.

   _____

4. Luckily, everything _____ _____ all right.

   _____

5. He was staring at me _____ _____ he knew me.

   _____

EXERCISES　**Word Order & Translation**　　CD 2-10 ▶ 50

日本文の意味に合うように，（　）内の語句を並べかえて英文を作りなさい。

1. 帰宅するまでには，私は本当に空腹だった。

   (I / really / got / the time / hungry / was / home / I / by).

   _____

2. 来週その問題を処理するための時間を作りましょう。

   (next week / with / to / make / the problem / deal / time / I'll).

   _____

3. ヘンリーは，日曜日は子どもたちと過ごすように努力している。

   (with / spending / a point / Henry / his children / Sundays / of / makes).

   _____

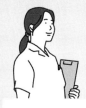

次の日本文の空欄に入る語を下から選びなさい。

> 自動体外式除細動器，　　手術室，　　主訴，　　心肺蘇生術，　　性感染症，
> 蘇生処置不要，　　点滴静脈，　　乳幼児突然死症候群

1. AED = automated external defibrillator

   AED is used to help those experiencing sudden cardiac arrest.

   _____ は，突然の心拍停止を経験している人を助けるのに使われる。

2. CC = chief complaint

   CC is the primary symptom that a patient states as the reason for seeking medical care.

   _____ とは，患者が医療を求める理由として述べる主な症状のことだ。

3. CPR = cardiopulmonary resuscitation

   CPR is an emergency lifesaving procedure performed when the heart stops beating.

   _____ は，心臓が停止した場合に行われる緊急の救命処置だ。

4. DNR = do not resuscitate

   A **DNR** order does not mean that no medical assistance will be given.

   _____ という指示は，医療支援を行わないということを意味するものではない。

5. IV = intravenous

   We learned how to start an **IV** drip.

   私たちは _____ 注射を始める方法を学んだ。

6. OR = operating room

   The baby was brought to the **OR** for excision of the tumor.

   その赤ちゃんは，腫瘍を切除するために _____ に運ばれた。

7. STD = sexually transmitted disease

   Chlamydia, gonorrhea, and herpes are **STDs**.

   クラミジア，淋病，ヘルペスは _____ だ。

8. SIDS = sudden infant death syndrome

   SIDS usually occurs when a baby is asleep.

   _____ は，ふつうは赤ちゃんが眠っている時に起こる。

Column

　医師や看護師が医療現場で何気なく使うことばによって，患者が傷ついたり，他の医療スタッフが勘違いしたりする場合があります。SOB という略語をめぐっては，患者が病院や医師を相手に訴訟を起こした例もあります。医師は患者の状態を説明するのに shortness of breath（息切れ，呼吸困難）の意味で使ったのですが，それを聞いた患者は，自分が son of a bitch（畜生）呼ばわりされたと思ったわけです。

　略語以外でも，看護師から vitals をとると言われた男性患者が激怒したとか，患者が arrest の状態になったと聞いた新人看護師が，その患者は何も悪いことをしていないと抗議したとか，患者のベッドサイドに stool を持ってきてほしいと頼んだだけなのに，必要のない検査をしそうになった，などのエピソードがあります。どんな勘違いが起きたのか，vitals，arrest，stool の 3 つの単語の意味を調べてみましょう。

Unit 11
Socks and All ...

An OR nurse opts for empathy and honesty in responding to an adolescent patient's fears.

* opt for ~　〜を選ぶ　　empathy　共感　　honesty　誠実　　adolescent　思春期の

Bryanne Hickey Harrington, BSN, RN, CNOR

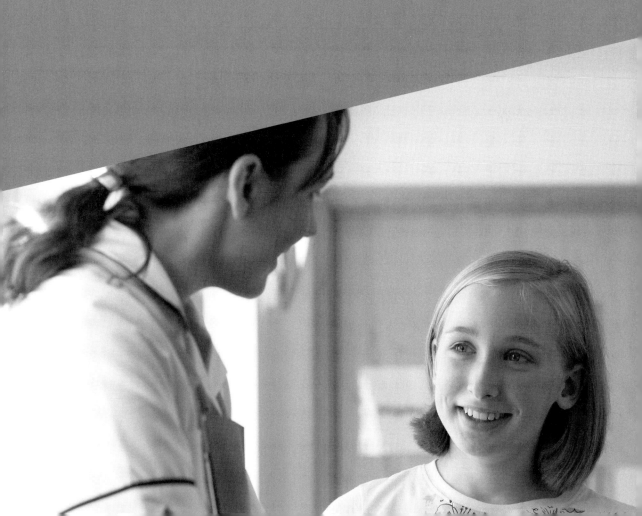

次の英語の意味に合う日本語を下から選びなさい。また，音声を聴いて発音しなさい。

1. tumor　　_____　　**2.** lesion　　_____

3. orthopedist　_____　　**4.** advocate　_____

5. modesty　　_____

整形外科医，擁護者，病変，慎み深さ，腫瘍

READING　**Essay【Part 1】**　　CD 2-12 ▶ 52

エッセイの出だしを読んでみましょう。

　　As the circulating nurse in our busy OR that Friday, I went to prepare our last case: "Katie," a 14-year-old who'd been diagnosed with multiple osteochondromas. These tumors are typically composed of bony fibers and cartilage. They're usually
5　benign but can cause pain. On several occasions Katie had come to the ED with pain so severe she'd vomited. She needed OxyContin to sleep at night and had stopped going to school. The lesion on the underside of her left arm was so painful she couldn't even brush her hair. A larger lesion on the inner aspect
10　of her scapula caused searing chest pain when she took a deep breath. She'd seen a neurologist, psychologists, the pain service, and finally our orthopedist, who would remove the lesions and give her back her life.

Medical and Nursing Notes

circulating nurse　外回り看護師
OR　手術室（operating room）
be diagnosed with ~　～と診断される
multiple　多発性の
osteochondroma　骨軟骨腫
bony　骨のような
fiber　線維
cartilage　軟骨，軟骨組織
benign　良性の（↔ malignant 悪性の）
ED　救急部門（emergency department）
vomit　吐く
OxyContin　（鎮痛薬の）オキシコンチン

scapula　肩甲骨
chest pain　胸痛
neurologist　神経科医
psychologist　心理学者
pain service　疼痛管理サービス

Notes　(l. 3) be composed of ~　～から成り立っている　　(l. 8) underside　裏側　　(l. 8) so ~ (that) ...　非常に～なので…
(l. 9) aspect　面　　(l. 10) searing　焼けつくような　　(l. 10) take a deep breath　深呼吸する
(l. 13) give A back B　A に B を取り戻させる

Check the situation

Q1　ブライアン（筆者）が金曜日最後に担当した手術患者が受けた診断は？

Q2　ケイティが深呼吸をすると胸に激しい痛みが生じる原因は？

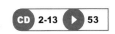

Medical and Nursing Notes

pre-op　手術前の（preoperative）

　　　　We were preparing the OR when the pre-op nurse called
to say Katie had locked herself in the bathroom and was crying
uncontrollably. Her mother was trying to talk to her through
the door. The problem was that Katie didn't want to remove
5　her bra—didn't want any men to see her naked. Her mother
wanted us to lie and say that the bra would stay on.

　　　　As a rule, an OR nurse's job is very technical; we interact
with patients and their families only briefly. Before the
operation we quickly assess the patient and ensure that she or
10　he is prepared for surgery. We introduce ourselves, then check
and double-check documents and lab results. Patients don't
often remember the nurses who hold their hands as they go
under anesthesia, nor do they realize that those nurses pride
themselves on being the patients' advocate while they're asleep.

surgery　手術

lab result　検査結果

go under anesthesia　麻酔がきく

15　　　　In the case of a pediatric patient, a parent or guardian
signs the consent forms. But if a child voices strong opposition to
surgery, it's the OR nurse's ethical responsibility to investigate
the concern. And so I assured Katie's mother that we'd take
excellent care of her daughter, but that I'd want to be honest in
20　speaking to Katie.

pediatric　小児科の

consent form　同意書

take care of ~　～の世話をする

　　　　I had to introduce myself to Katie through the bathroom
door. Once she let me in, I gave her a tissue and asked her to sit
down and take a deep breath. I told her I'd explain everything
that was going to happen from the time we left the pre-op area,
25　and that it was my job to keep her safe through her surgery.
I said I'd answer her questions. I said I wanted her to feel
comfortable with the plan before we went ahead.

　　　　Katie responded that she wouldn't take off her bra and
didn't want anyone to see her naked. As I crouched in front of
30　her, I thought how much easier it would be to do as her mother

had asked and just lie. But I knew this would violate Katie's modesty, and the trust she'd just put in me. I didn't want to fuel a distrust of those who'd care for her in the future. And I remembered how difficult it was to be 14, with raging emotions
5 and a changing body.

So I told Katie the truth: eventually, the bra had to come off.

At first, she seemed even more upset. But then I told her I'd be the one to take the bra off after she was asleep—the one keeping her covered, making sure only those who needed to
10 be there were there. I promised to treat her like I'd want to be treated myself. And that all this would be worth it not to have the horrible pain.

Katie was still crying when I said the surgeon would be coming to see her in a few minutes. I told her I'd watch the
15 bathroom door from the outside if she kept it unlocked. I told her to think about what I'd said. Then I went to inform the attending surgeon about the mother's concerns and Katie's wishes.

At last, Katie emerged from the bathroom, her eyes
20 swollen, nose dripping. She said she'd do it if it would happen as I told her it would.

We proceeded. After several hours, two osteochondromas the size of golf balls had been removed. Before Katie woke up, I redressed her—socks and all—and wheeled her to the postanes-
25 thesia area. I went to visit her that following Monday. She told me she was embarrassed that she'd cried but was glad I'd told her the truth.

In the perioperative area it's easy to forget the value of simple actions like preserving the modesty of our patients. But
30 on this day, communicating honestly with my patient paved the way for a successful surgery.

care for ~   ~の世話をする

surgeon   外科医

attending   担当の, 主治医の

wheel   （ストレッチャーなどに乗せて）運ぶ
postanesthesia   麻酔後の

perioperative   周術期の, 手術前後の

Notes (l. 1) violate   背く   (l. 3) fuel   あおりたてる   (l. 3) distrust   不信感   (l. 3) those who ~   ~する人たち
(l. 4) raging   猛烈な   (l. 6) come off   はずれる   (l. 7) at first   最初は
(l. 9) make sure ~   間違いなく~するようにする   (l. 11) worth it   それだけの価値がある
(l. 12) horrible   ぞっとするほど嫌な   (l. 19) at last   ついに, ようやく   (l. 19) emerge   出てくる
(l. 22) proceed   先へ進む   (l. 24) redress   再び着せる   (l. 26) embarrassed   きまりの悪い思いをした
(l. 29) preserve   保つ   (l. 30) pave the way for ~   ~への道を開く, ~を可能にする

70

Reading Comprehension

次の英文が，本文の内容と一致する場合は T，一致しない場合は F を選びなさい。

1. (T / F) Katie didn't come out of the bathroom because she didn't want to have surgery.
2. (T / F) Katie's mother wanted Bryanne to tell the truth to Katie.
3. (T / F) Patients forget the nurses who held their hands as they were put under anesthesia.
4. (T / F) Bryanne didn't wanted anyone to remove Katie's bra.
5. (T / F) Katie was glad because Bryanne was honest in speaking to her.

EXERCISES **Dictation & Translation** CD 2-14 ▶ 54

音声を聴いて英文の空欄に適語を記入しなさい。また，完成した英文を日本語に直しなさい。

1. The patient _____ _____ _____ _____ .

   _____

2. Who will _____ _____ _____ the children?

   _____

3. They were sitting _____ _____ _____ me.

   _____

4. _____ _____ , I thought she was joking.

   _____

5. _____ _____, they were able to afford a house.

   _____

EXERCISES **Word Order & Translation** CD 2-15 ▶ 55

日本文の意味に合うように，（ ） 内の語句を並べかえて英文を作りなさい。

1. 問題は多くの生徒が朝食抜きで登校するということだ。

   (school / many students / the problem / without / come / is / eating / to / that / breakfast).

   _____

2. 私たちは仕事の質を誇りにしている。

   (our work / the quality / ourselves / we / of / on / pride).

   _____

3. その交渉によってさらなるビジネスへの道が開かれるはずだ。

   (should / business / for / pave / the negotiation / more / the way).

   _____

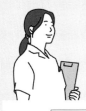

Nursing Terms and Expressions

次の日本文の空欄に入る語を下から選びなさい。

おむつ，　ガーゼ，　吸入器，　血圧計，　除細動器，　注射器，　包帯，　メス

---

1. The paramedics shocked her with a **defibrillator** and performed CPR for a further two minutes.
   救急救命士たちは＿＿＿＿＿＿＿＿で電気ショックを与えて，さらに 2 分間心肺蘇生術を行った。

2. The baby was wearing a disposable **diaper**.
   その赤ちゃんは，使い捨ての＿＿＿＿＿＿＿＿をつけていた。

3. The nurse came to change his **dressing**.
   看護師が彼の＿＿＿＿＿＿＿＿を交換するためにやってきた。

4. The nurse covered the cut with a piece of **gauze**.
   看護師は，その切り傷を＿＿＿＿＿＿＿＿で覆った。

5. People with asthma may need to use their **inhaler** every day.
   喘息の人は，＿＿＿＿＿＿＿＿を毎日使う必要があるかもしれない。

6. **Scalpels** are used by surgeons during operations.
   ＿＿＿＿＿＿＿＿は手術中に外科医が使用する。

7. A **sphygmomanometer** is an instrument for measuring blood pressure.
   ＿＿＿＿＿＿＿＿は，血圧を測定するための器具だ。

8. The nurse took a sample of my blood in a **syringe**.
   看護師は，＿＿＿＿＿＿＿＿で血液サンプルを採った。

Column

　米国の場合，paramedic は，EMS（Emergency Medical Service）と呼ばれる緊急医療サービスを行う医療専門職 EMT（Emergency Medical Technician）のなかでも最もレベルが高い EMT-Paramedic のことです。日本の「救急救命士」に近いものです。この paramedic や EMT が乗って出動するのが ambulance（救急車）ですが，そのフロント部分には ᗺƆИA⅃UᗺMA と表示されているのをよく見かけます。前を走っている車のドライバーがバックミラー（rearview mirror）越しに見ると，後方から AMBULANCE が接近していることがわかるようになっています。

　さて，米国の病院前に CABULANCE と書かれた車両が駐車していることがありますが，辞書には出てこない単語です。緊急を要しない患者を病院から別の病院へ，あるいは自宅へ移送する場合などに使用されます。この単語はどのような成り立ちでできているか考えてみましょう。

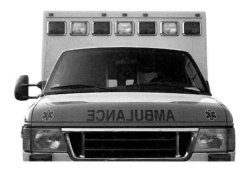

Unit 12

The Dirtiest House in Town

Home care nursing isn't for the faint of heart.

* faint of heart　臆病な人

Alice C. Facente, MSN, RN-BC

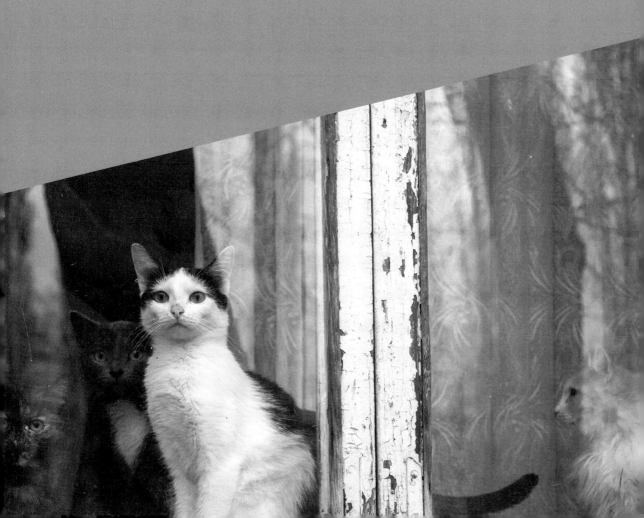

次の英語の意味に合う日本語を下から選びなさい。また，音声を聴いて発音しなさい。

1. referral _____ 2. diabetes _____

3. urine _____ 4. prescription _____

5. utensil _____

台所用品，尿，紹介状，処方薬，糖尿病

READING　**Essay【Part 1】**　CD 2-17 ▶ 57

エッセイの出だしを読んでみましょう。

Medical and Nursing Notes

convalescent-home　回復期施設,
病後療養所
stroke　脳卒中

discharge planner　（退院の計画を
立てる）ケアマネジャー
home care　在宅ケア

admitting nurse　入所担当看護師

take care of ~　～の世話をする

personal physician　かかりつけ医

911　（米国で警察・救急車・消防
車を呼ぶための）緊急電話番号

　　　The convalescent-home referral said that Loretta was 71 years old with the usual health problems related to stroke and diabetes. It also said that her husband had a gun and "wasn't afraid to use it." Fiercely protective of his wife, he'd had many
5 disputes with the nursing staff about her care. The discharge planner who'd referred her to our home care agency insisted that two nurses make the initial home visit.

　　　When I arrived at the home, the admitting nurse was already in the driveway, embroiled in a discussion with the
10 husband. Insisting that he'd take care of Loretta himself, he refused to allow us in the house. Although we told him that his wife's personal physician, whom he claimed to trust, had asked for our help, he remained adamant. Finally, after I said that we'd have to call 911 for a police escort, he let us in.

Notes　(l. 4) fiercely　猛烈に　　(l. 4) protective of ~　～を保護したがる　　(l. 5) dispute　言い争い，口論
(l. 6) refer　紹介する　　(l. 9) driveway　（通りから玄関までの）私道　　(l. 9) embroiled　巻き込まれて
(l. 12) ask for ~　～を求める，～を頼む　　(l. 13) adamant　断固として譲らない　　(l. 14) police escort　警護
(l. 14) let ~ in　～を中に入れる

Check the situation

Q1　ロレッタの夫と看護師たちとの関係は？

Q2　ロレッタの自宅を訪問した 2 人の看護師が最後に取った手段は？

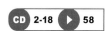
An overpowering odor of urine hit us as we entered the living room. We soon discovered it was from the couple's 14 cats and two dogs. The litter box was overflowing. It was so dark and dirty inside the house, we couldn't tell if the floor was

5 linoleum or wood.

Loretta was sitting on the edge of a hospital bed in the living room, smiling. We introduced ourselves and told her we were there to take care of her. "I'm so happy to be home," she said, hugging her husband and two of the nearest cats. With

10 her husband hovering nearby, we began a complete physical assessment.

> physical assessment　フィジカルア
> セスメント（問診などの身体診査
> 技術を用いて健康上の問題を評価
> すること）
> fill　処方する

Her husband had all of her prescriptions filled and purchased an alternating air pressure mattress for the hospital bed, three sets of bed linens, pads for the bed, and an

15 assortment of incontinence briefs.

> alternating air pressure mattress
> （褥瘡予防に使う）交互空気圧マッ
> トレス
> bed linen　ベッド用シーツと枕カ
> バー
> incontinence brief　失禁用のブ
> リーフ
> Meals on Wheels　ミールズ・オン・
> ホイールズ（老人や病人に対する
> 食事の宅配サービス）

We offered the services of Meals on Wheels, but he refused. The kitchen counters were grimy and cluttered. The kitchen sink was plugged, full of black, stagnant water and greasy pots. The only thing on the large wooden table was an aluminum

20 baking pan filled with dry cat food. A cat lounged on every flat surface: the kitchen cabinets, counters, hospital bed, even the wheelchair. We didn't try to reason with the couple about sanitation issues surrounding these pets, at least not on this first visit.

> wheelchair　車椅子
>
> sanitation　衛生

25 We gave Loretta a sponge bath with her husband watching our every move. We taught him how to empty the urinary drainage bag and monitor her blood sugar, and instructed him on her medications, simplifying procedures wherever possible.

> give ~ a sponge bath　～を清拭す
> る
> urinary drainage bag　採尿バッグ
>
> blood sugar　血糖
>
> medication　投薬

Each step of the way, we praised him for his fast learning.
30 We told him we appreciated how devoted he was to Loretta,

otes (l. 1) overpowering　非常に強い　　(l. 1) odor　におい　　(l. 3) litter box　猫用トイレ　　(l. 3) overflow　溢れる
(l. 5) linoleum　リノリウム　　(l. 10) hover　うろうろする　　(l. 13) purchase　購入する
(l. 15) assortment　（同一物を）各種集めたもの　　(l. 17) grimy　汚れた　　(l. 17) cluttered　散らかった
(l. 18) plugged　詰まった　　(l. 18) stagnant　よどんだ　　(l. 18) greasy　脂で汚れた　　(l. 18) pot　丸く深い容器
(l. 20) baking pan　焼き型　　(l. 20) lounge　ゆったり横になる　　(l. 22) reason with ~　～を説得する
(l. 23) at least　少なくとも　　(l. 28) simplify　簡単にする　　(l. 30) appreciate　高く評価する
(l. 30) devoted　献身的な

Unit 12　The Dirtiest House in Town　**75**

and that our goal was to help him continue to take good care of her. Loretta seemed oblivious to the dirty environment and her husband's intimidating manner, and accepted all of the care we provided.

5　　By the time we were ready to leave, he hugged us, thanked us, and said we could come back anytime.

　　During my visit the next day, I convinced him to allow a home health aide to come and bathe Loretta. He agreed—but only if I made my nursing visits at the same time. When I
10　arrived for the third visit, the husband showed me how he had unclogged the toilet, mopped the kitchen floor, and thrown all the dirty dishes in the garbage; he bought paper plates and plastic utensils to use.

　　The house never became what could be described as
15　clean, but Loretta and her clothing always were. Loretta never developed pressure ulcers, pneumonia, or deep vein thrombosis. She had frequent urinary tract infections from the indwelling catheter, but her husband phoned me immediately when he recognized signs of infection, just as I had taught him.

20　　At the end of every visit he always thanked me, and I never did see that legendary gun.

home health aide （在宅介護をする）在宅ケア助手，在宅介護士
bathe 入浴させる

pressure ulcer 褥瘡
pneumonia 肺炎
deep vein thrombosis 深部静脈血栓症
urinary tract infection 尿路感染症
indwelling catheter 留置カテーテル

Notes　(l. 2) oblivious　気づかない　　(l. 3) intimidating　威嚇するような　　(l. 5) by the time ~　～する時までには
(l. 5) be ready to ~　～する準備ができている　　(l. 7) convince A to ~　A に～するよう説得する
(l. 9) only if ~　～する場合に限り　　(l. 9) at the same time　同時に　　(l. 11) unclog　障害物を取り除く
(l. 12) garbage　ごみ集積所　　(l. 20) at the end of ~　～の終わりに　　(l. 21) legendary　有名な

Reading Comprehension

次の英文が，本文の内容と一致する場合は T，一致しない場合は F を選びなさい。

1. (T / F) The two nurses made the home visit because Loretta's husband had a gun.

2. (T / F) The nurses reasoned with Loretta and his husband about sanitation issues surrounding their cats and dogs.

3. (T / F) The nurses taught Loretta's husband how to give her a sponge bath.

4. (T / F) When the nurse arrived for the third visit, the house was cleaner than before.

5. (T / F) As soon as Loretta's husband recognized signs of infection, he called the nurse.

音声を聴いて英文の空欄に適語を記入しなさい。また，完成した英文を日本語に直しなさい。

1. She _____ _____ a cup of tea.

   _____

2. She unlocked the door and _____ me _____.

   _____

3. It's no use to _____ _____ him.

   _____

4. I can't concentrate on two things _____ _____
   _____ _____.

   _____

5. I'm going on vacation _____ _____ _____
   _____ September.

   _____

日本文の意味に合うように，（ ）内の語句を並べかえて英文を作りなさい。

1. 私たちは新生児の沐浴方法を学んだ。

   (a sponge bath / give / how / we / a newborn / to / learned).

   _____

2. スーザンは一緒に暮らすよう祖父を説得することを試みた。

   (her / live / her grandfather / to / Susan / with / to / convince / tried).

   _____

3. 非常時のみこのドアを使用できる。

   (use / we / is / if / this door / can / an emergency / there / only).

   _____

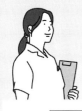

Nursing Terms and Expressions

次の日本文の空欄に入る語を下から選びなさい。

肝炎，　骨折，　骨粗しょう症，　統合失調症，　捻挫，　白血病

---

1. He sustained multiple **fractures** in a motorcycle accident.
オートバイ事故の後，彼は多発性＿＿＿＿＿＿＿＿を負った。

2. **Hepatitis** is a serious disease which affects the liver.
＿＿＿＿＿＿＿＿は，肝臓に影響を与える重い病気だ。

3. Several new treatment options for **leukemia** are currently under development.
＿＿＿＿＿＿＿＿に対するいくつかの新しい治療の選択肢は，現在開発中だ。

4. Women are much more likely to develop **osteoporosis** than men.
女性は，男性よりもはるかに＿＿＿＿＿＿＿＿を発症しやすい。

5. She continued to play despite an ankle **sprain**.
足首の＿＿＿＿＿＿＿＿にもかかわらず，彼女はプレーを続けた。

6. He was diagnosed with **schizophrenia**.
彼は＿＿＿＿＿＿＿＿だと診断された。

Column

　hepatitis = *hepat-*（「肝臓」の意味の連結形） + *-itis*（「…炎」の意味の接尾辞）です。 *-itis* を含む bronchitis と gastritis の意味とその単語の成り立ちを調べてみましょう。

　leukemia = *leuk-*（「白血球」の意味の連結形） + *-emia*（「血液中に…を有する状態」の連結形）です。 *-emia* を含む bacteremia と uremia の意味と単語の成り立ちを調べてみましょう。

　osteoporosis = *osteo-*（「骨」の意味の連結形） + *por-*（「孔」の意味の連結形） + *-osis*（「…病，…症」の意味の接尾辞）です。 *-osis* を含む neurosis と tuberculosis の意味と単語の成り立ちを調べてみましょう。

　さて，adenoma（腺腫）や sarcoma（肉腫）に使われている *-oma* は「腫，溜」の意味ですが，医療現場ではこの連結形 *-oma* を使った，辞書には出てこない単語が使われることがあります。例えば，fascinoma は *fascinating*（「魅惑的な」） + *-oma* からできた語で，医師にとって興味をそそる病気や患者のことです。逆に興味のないものは unfascinoma です。また，horrendioma は *horrendous*（「恐ろしい」） + *-oma* からできた語で，恐ろしいほど悪い症状とか恐ろしく大きな腫瘍などを指して使われます。

Unit 13

Hiding a Tender Soul

*tender　思いやりのある

A cold day on the waterfront, a nurse, a homeless man, and a canary yellow coat.

* waterfront　海岸地区　　canary yellow　カナリア色

Cheryl Kane, MEd, BSN, RN

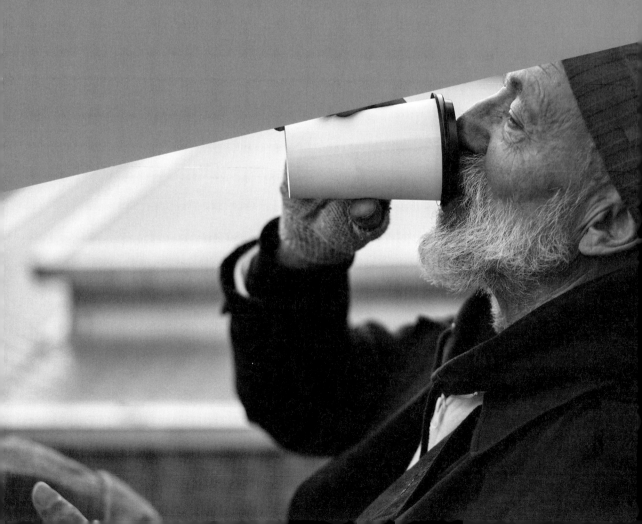

次の英語の意味に合う日本語を下から選びなさい。また，音声を聴いて発音しなさい。

1. neighborhood _____

2. divorce _____

3. complexion _____

4. disconcert _____

5. generous _____

寛容な，顔色，地域，困惑させる，離婚

READING   **Essay 【Part 1】**   CD 2-22 ▶ 62

エッセイの出だしを読んでみましょう。

Medical and Nursing Notes

Patrick had once been a fisherman, living in Boston's North End, a predominantly Italian neighborhood until the young professionals moved in and many old-timers moved out. He had been married and gainfully employed before his life spiraled
5 out of control and his low self-esteem, gambling, and drinking resulted in divorce and homelessness.

Patrick was disheveled, dirty, alcoholic, and feisty, although he could be a real charmer. Seventy years old, he was slight of build with a ruddy complexion, a bushy gray beard, and long,
10 dirty fingernails.

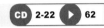
alcoholic　アルコール依存症の

fingernail　指のつめ

Notes
(l. 1) fisherman　漁師　　(l. 1) North End　ノースエンド（米国マサチューセッツ州ボストン北部のイタリア人街）
(l. 2) predominantly　圧倒的に，主に　　(l. 3) old-timer　老人　　(l. 4) gainfully　有給で　　(l. 4) spiral　悪化する
(l. 5) out of control　制しきれなくなって　　(l. 5) self-esteem　自尊心　　(l. 6) result in ~　〜の結果になる
(l. 6) homelessness　家のない状態　　(l. 7) disheveled　（髪が）ぼさぼさの，（服装が）だらしない
(l. 7) feisty　威勢のいい　　(l. 8) charmer　魅力のある人　　(l. 8) slight　きゃしゃな　　(l. 9) build　体格
(l. 9) ruddy　血色のよい　　(l. 9) bushy　もじゃもじゃの　　(l. 9) beard　あごひげ

Check the situation

Q1　パトリックが離婚してホームレスになった原因3つは？

Q2　パトリックの外見は？

Medical and Nursing Notes

Patrick hung out near the New England Aquarium next to the harbor. He spent his days stemming—street slang for panhandling. In the evening, he slept between Jersey barriers on a busy street that traces the shape of Boston's shoreline. In
5　cold weather, he would wrap himself in the dark gray, felt-like blankets homeless advocates hand out when the temperatures drop.

advocate　擁護者，支持者

As a member of the Boston Health Care for the Homeless Program's street team, I had been his nurse for several years.
10　I knew the outlines of his early life: his mother died young; his stepmother rejected him. He often talked about killing himself. I once asked Patrick if he was scared to die and he told me that even God wouldn't want him. He rarely accepted health care from our team, but occasionally would allow us to take him
15　back to one of the shelters for a shower and change of clothes.

Boston Health Care for the Homeless Program　ホームレスのためのボストン保健医療プログラム（略称はBHCHP で，1985 年発足）

One fall day, Patrick had been lying on a wall that ran along Boston Harbor when a friend pushed him into the water. He suffered a massive coronary and was hospitalized. A few weeks later I got a page from the local hospital, saying Patrick
20　had left the hospital against doctor's orders, wearing only a hospital johnny and a vest.

suffer　（苦痛などを）経験する
massive　（病気が）組織の広範囲に及ぶ
coronary　心臓発作（heart attack）
hospitalize　入院させる

johnny　患者用ガウン

It was an unusually cold Sunday in October. I rushed out to look for him. I wasn't surprised to find him in his usual spot between the Jersey barriers, swathed in blankets. I led him
25　across the street and asked him to wait in front of the Dunkin' Donuts while I went to get him some clothes. When I returned with a set of men's clothes and a canary yellow down jacket, Patrick looked at me, then glanced disdainfully at the jacket and

Notes
(l. 1) hang out　住む　　(l. 1) New England Aquarium　ニューイングランド水族館　　(l. 1) next to ~　〜の隣の
(l. 2) spend 時間 ~ing　〜して時間を過ごす　　(l. 2) stem　ねだる，たかる　　(l. 3) panhandle　街頭で物乞いをする
(l. 3) Jersey barrier　ジャージーバリア，コンクリート防護柵（米国ニュージャージー州の幹線道路用に開発されたことに由来）
(l. 4) trace　なぞる，たどる　　(l. 4) shoreline　海岸線　　(l. 5) felt-like　フェルト状の　　(l. 6) hand out　配る
(l. 11) stepmother　継母　　(l. 11) kill oneself　自殺する　　(l. 12) be scared to ~　〜するのが怖い
(l. 13) rarely ~　めったに〜しない　　(l. 14) occasionally　ときおり　　(l. 14) allow A to ~　A が〜するのを許す
(l. 17) Boston Harbor　ボストン港　　(l. 19) page　呼び出し　　(l. 23) look for ~　〜をさがす　　(l. 24) swathe　包む
(l. 25) in front of ~　〜の前で　　(l. 25) Dunkin' Donuts　ダンキンドーナッツ　　(l. 28) glance at ~　〜をちらっと見る
(l. 28) disdainfully　軽蔑的に

said that if he wore it, he would stick out like a sore thumb. He asked me where in the world I had gotten it.

I told him that it had belonged to my husband, Jim. When he asked me if he no longer wanted it, I told him Jim had died two years ago and would have been very happy for him to use it. Patrick's demeanor softened. "Oh, honey. I'm so sorry. Go into that Dunkin' Donuts, buy yourself a coffee—put it on my tab," he instructed. "Then come back and tell me all about your husband."

I went into Dunkin' Donuts and bought a coffee. I paid for it myself. When I returned, he invited me to sit on a milk crate and tell him about my husband. I told him how we hadn't been married for very long before Jim developed a brain tumor, how sick he had gotten, how he loved to run marathons. What I didn't tell Patrick was that our wedding anniversary was that weekend. It was always a difficult time of year for me. My moments of connection with Patrick made it a little easier.

brain tumor　脳腫瘍

That encounter with Patrick shaped my nursing practice. Working with long-term homeless people can be very challenging, physically and emotionally. Their lice-infested bodies can disconcert even the most experienced nurse. Cleaning them can take your breath away. They can be rejecting, belligerent, ungrateful.

lice-infested　シラミだらけの

Yet here was this homeless man who fit every stereotype, reaching out to me at a time when I was very vulnerable. His generous spirit and sensitivity taught me the importance of looking beyond the exterior. The tenderest of souls can be contained within the most unlikely of vessels. You just have to take a moment to look.

Our patients have been victims of emotional, sexual, and physical violence. Their ability to trust is limited. When a patient trusts us enough to tell us who they really are, it is a sacred moment.

Notes (l. 1) stick out like a sore thumb　場違いである　　(l. 2) in the world　（疑問詞を強調して）一体全体
(l. 4) no longer ~　もはや~ではない　　(l. 6) demeanor　態度　　(l. 8) tab　勘定書，伝票　　(l. 12) crate　ケース
(l. 18) encounter　出会い　　(l. 19) work with ~　~を相手に働く　　(l. 22) take A's breath away　A の息をのませる
(l. 23) belligerent　けんか腰の　　(l. 23) ungrateful　感謝をしていない　　(l. 24) stereotype　固定観念，既成概念
(l. 25) reach out to ~　~と心を通わせる　　(l. 25) vulnerable　傷つきやすい　　(l. 26) sensitivity　思いやり
(l. 27) exterior　外面　　(l. 28) vessel　器　　(l. 33) sacred　聖なる

Reading Comprehension

次の英文が，本文の内容と一致する場合はT，一致しない場合はFを選びなさい。

1. (T / F) Patrick lived near the New England Aquarium next to Boston's North End.
2. (T / F) Patrick often accepted health care from Boston Health Care for the Homeless Program.
3. (T / F) Patrick thought that if he wore the canary yellow jacket he would look out of place.
4. (T / F) After Patrick bought a coffee for Cheryl (the writer), she told him about her husband.
5. (T / F) Working with homeless people required considerable physical and emotional effort.

EXERCISES **Dictation & Translation** CD 2-24 ▶ 64

音声を聴いて英文の空欄に適語を記入しなさい。また，完成した英文を日本語に直しなさい。

1. The crash _____ _____ the deaths of 23 passengers.

   _____

2. My father sat down _____ _____ me without a word.

   _____

3. Everyone _____ too _____ _____ move.

   _____

4. George _____ _____ his watch.

   _____

5. She _____ _____ plays in the orchestra.

   _____

EXERCISES **Word Order & Translation** CD 2-25 ▶ 65

日本文の意味に合うように，（ ）内の語句を並べかえて英文を作りなさい。

1. 彼女たちは週末の大半を使ってナースステーションをきれいにした。

   (the nurses' station / cleaning / of / spent / up / the weekend / most / they).

   _____

2. 彼女の両親は彼女が夜遊びすることを許さないだろう。

   (to / late / stay / her / won't / out / allow / her parents).

   _____

3. いったいなぜ私があなたの話に耳を傾けなけなければならないの？

   (you / listen / should / in / to / I / the world / why)?

   _____

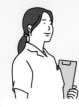

Nursing Terms and Expressions

次の英文と日本文を参考にして，空欄に英語を記入しなさい

1. ADL = activities of _____ living
   How quickly **ADL**s are regained after a heart attack varies from person to person.
   心臓発作後にどれくらい早く**日常生活動作**が回復するかは，人によって異なる。

2. CDC = Centers for _____ Control and Prevention
   The **CDC** was founded in 1946 as the Communicable Disease Center.
   （米国）**疾病対策センター**は，伝染病センターとして 1946 年に設立された。

3. ECG = _____ cardiogram
   Your doctor may suggest you get an **ECG** to check for signs of heart disease.
   主治医は，心臓疾患の徴候を調べるために**心電図**をとるよう提案するかもしれない。

4. ENT = ear, nose, and _____
   The **ENT** doctor said her nosebleeds were nothing to worry about.
   その**耳鼻咽喉科**医は，彼女の鼻血は何も心配することはないと言った。

5. PTSD = post-traumatic stress _____
   PTSD is a condition that occurs after experiencing or witnessing a traumatic event.
   心的外傷後ストレス障害は，悲惨な出来事を経験したり目撃したりした後に起こる状態だ。

6. QOL = _____ of life
   QOL is a major concern of patients with terminal cancer.
   生活の質は，末期がん患者の大きな関心だ。

7. RDS = respiratory distress _____
   RDS occurs in premature babies whose lungs are not fully developed.
   呼吸窮迫症候群は，肺が十分発達していない未熟児で起こる。

8. WHO = World Health _____
   The **WHO** was established in 1948 as a specialized agency of the United Nations.
   世界保健機関は，国際連合の専門機関として 1948 年に設立された。

Column

　attention deficit hyperactivity disorder（注意欠陥多動性障害）の頭文字 ADHD は，アルファベットを一文字ずつ「エイ・ディー・エイチ・ディー」と読みます。一方で acquired immune deficiency [immunodeficiency] syndrome（後天性免疫不全症候群）の頭文字 AIDS は，ひとつの単語のように「エイズ」と読みます。後者のような略語を acronym（頭字語）と呼びます。

　intensive care unit（集中治療室）の頭文字 ICU は「アイ・シー・ユー」ですが，医療現場では，その前に neonatal がつく neonatal intensive care unit（新生児集中治療室）の頭文字 NICU は「ニック・ユー」，surgical がつく surgical intensive care unit（外科集中治療室）の頭文字 SICU は「シック・ユー」のように読むことも多いようです。次のように読む略語の意味を調べてみましょう。

1. 「キャット」　= CAT (computerized [computed] axial tomography)
2. 「ポッド」　　= POD (post operative day)
3. 「ライス」　　= RICE (rest, ice, compression, elevation)
4. 「キャベッジ」= CABG (coronary artery bypass graft)
5. 「エンセッド」= NSAID (nonsteroidal anti-inflammatory drug)

Unit 14

Keeping Secrets

A nurse remembers the cost—to both patients and herself—
of keeping silent about AIDS.

* cost 犠牲，代償

Elena Schwolsky, MPH, RN

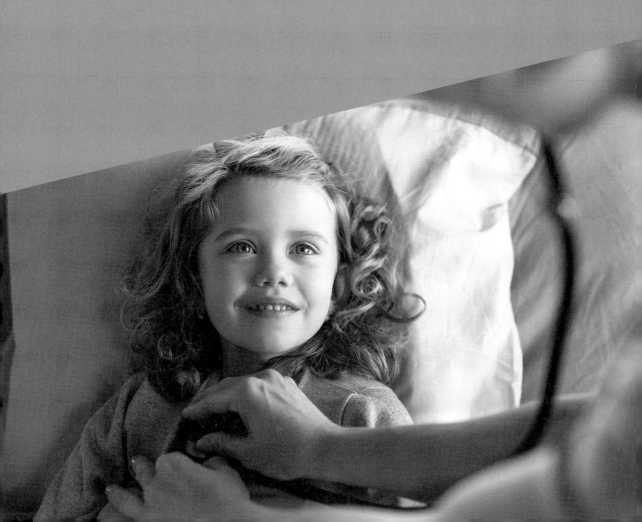

次の英語の意味に合う日本語を下から選びなさい。また，音声を聴いて発音しなさい。

1. reluctance _____   **2.** diagnosis _____

3. guilt _____   **4.** funeral _____

5. diminish _____

診断，減少する，罪悪感，気が進まないこと，葬儀

READING   Essay【Part 1】

CD 2-27 ▶ 67

エッセイの出だしを読んでみましょう。

Medical and Nursing Notes

In the spring of 1988, two months after my husband, Clarence, was diagnosed with AIDS, I went to work as a pediatric AIDS nurse at a clinic in New Jersey. Clarence had fought in Vietnam, and now he was on the front lines of this
5　epidemic. I felt a need to be there too. It was a time when treatment options ran out fast. The kids I cared for got very sick and soon died. Activists were marching in the streets with signs proclaiming "Silence = Death," but for many, AIDS was something to be whispered about or not spoken of at all. I
10　became a keeper of secrets, and one of them was my own.

"I don't want everyone to see me as your husband who has AIDS, babe," Clarence said. "I want them to know me first as a person, not a disease." I was puzzled—my never-shy husband could get up in a crowded 12-step meeting and declare, "Hi, I'm
15　Clarence and I'm an addict." Why this reluctance? We argued about it, but in the end agreed we'd tell only close friends and family.

be diagnosed with ~　～と診断される
AIDS　エイズ，後天性免疫不全症候群（acquired immunodeficiency syndrome）
pediatric　小児科の
epidemic　流行病

treatment　治療
care for ~　～の世話をする

12-step　（依存症脱却プログラムが）12段階からなる
addict　（麻薬などの）常用者

Notes

(l. 3) New Jersey　米国ニュージャージー州　　(l. 6) run out　尽きる　　(l. 7) activist　活動家
(l. 8) proclaim　宣言する　　(l. 9) whisper about ~　～についてうわさ話をする　　(l. 9) not ~ at all　全然～でない
(l. 9) speak of ~　～について語る　　(l. 11) see A as B　A を B とみなす　　(l. 12) babe　（夫婦間の呼びかけで）おまえ
(l. 13) puzzled　困惑した　　(l. 13) never-shy　決して恥ずかしがらない　　(l. 16) in the end　結局

Check the situation

Q1　1988 年当時，エイズ治療はどのような状況だったか？

Q2　エレナ（筆者）とクラレンスが話し合って出した結論は？

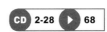

Medical and Nursing Notes

Each day I carried my secret to work, where the families I cared for were also hesitant to mention their child's diagnosis. A combination of shame and fear had driven some halfway across the state to avoid being seen in an AIDS clinic in their

5 hometowns. The stigma was intense, even for children, who were considered "innocent" victims. On the nightly news we saw images of a tearful Ryan White, barred from attending school, and a frightened family in Florida burned out of their home. But everyone had their own worries about public

10 disclosure, their own stories to conceal.

There was a child I'll never forget—Jasmine, one of the sickest on my case-load, a bright eight-year-old with a wise little face framed by frizzy brown hair. She lived with her mother and grandmother, but was often in the hospital. I'd usually

15 find her on a comfortably padded stretcher next to the nurses' station.

Concerned that Jasmine might overhear a careless remark on the ward, the social worker and I tried to persuade her mother to tell her that she had AIDS. But Jasmine's mother

20 refused to even discuss it. Perhaps she couldn't bear the guilt over having transmitted the virus to Jasmine. I longed to move beyond the labels that separated us—nurse, wife, mother, person with AIDS—and share my own story. But I kept my promise to Clarence.

25 One day, as we made rounds, I found Jasmine at her usual post. Pale and listless, with barely enough energy to create another of the crayon drawings that decorated our cubicles, she called me over. "I want to talk to you about something

nurses' station　ナースステーション

ward　病棟
social worker　ソーシャルワーカー

transmit　伝染させる

make rounds　巡回する

Notes (l. 2) be hesitant to ~　~するのをためらう　　(l. 3) halfway　ある程度, かなり　　(l. 4) state　州
(l. 5) stigma　汚名　　(l. 6) nightly　毎晩の　　(l. 7) tearful　涙ぐんだ
(l. 7) Ryan White　ライアン・ホワイト (1971-1990)　エイズに感染したために学校から追放され18歳で亡くなった少年
(l. 7) bar A from ~ing　Aが~することを禁止する　　(l. 8) frightened　怯えた
(l. 8) Florida　米国フロリダ州　　(l. 8) burned out of ~　~から焼け出された　　(l. 9) public disclosure　開示
(l. 10) conceal　隠す　　(l. 12) case-load　担当件数　　(l. 12) bright　利口な　　(l. 13) frame　縁をつける
(l. 13) frizzy　縮れ毛の　　(l. 15) padded　詰め物の入った　　(l. 15) next to ~　~の隣の
(l. 17) overhear　ふと耳にする　　(l. 17) remark　発言　　(l. 18) persuade A to ~　Aを説得して~させる
(l. 20) bear　耐える　　(l. 21) long to ~　~したいと切望する　　(l. 26) post　持ち場　　(l. 26) listless　元気のない
(l. 26) barely　かろうじて　　(l. 27) cubicle　小部屋　　(l. 28) call ~ over　~を呼び寄せる

important," she said, obviously making an effort to talk. I prepared myself. Was she going to ask me the question I couldn't answer? Wasn't I bound to respect her mother's wishes?

I leaned over Jasmine's stretcher to hear. "I am very sick,"
5 she whispered, pausing for breath. "I think I have AIDS. But you have to promise. Don't tell my mother. It's a secret … She would be sad if she found out."

A few weeks later, at Jasmine's funeral, I wondered if she and her mother had found a way to speak honestly before she
10 died. And again I wished I could have let her mother know how much I shared in her pain.

Clarence died a year later after a long slide, and I no longer had to keep silent. Only then did I begin to acknowledge my own fears. At the bereavement support group, when it was time to
15 share my own story, I "passed," afraid the cancer widows would judge me. For years afterward, when someone would innocently ask, "How did your husband die?" the answer would stick in my throat. I found myself carefully measuring the questioner: Would they ask how he got it?—AIDS always seems to raise that
20 question. And how would they feel about me if they knew?

It's been more than 15 years since I left my job at the clinic. Times have changed and the stigma has diminished. Meanwhile, the incidence of AIDS is on the rise again, particularly among young women of color. I think of the
25 thousands who will be diagnosed this year, and wonder if they will suffer alone, afraid to speak.

The secret I kept for Clarence still has power over me. Even now, when a new acquaintance asks about my late husband, I hesitate. Then I remember Jasmine and that painful silence we
30 all kept back then. I take a breath, and speak in a clear, strong voice: "My husband died of AIDS."

bereavement　死別
support group　（共通の悩みや経験をもち支えあう）サポートグループ
cancer　がん

incidence　発生（率）

die of ~　～が原因で死ぬ

Notes　(l. 1) make an effort to ~　～しようと努力する　　(l. 2) prepare oneself　覚悟をする
(l. 3) be bound to ~　～する責任がある　　(l. 4) lean over ~　～の上にかがみこむ
(l. 5) pause for breath　息をつく　　(l. 7) find out　事実を知る　　(l. 8) wonder if ~　～かどうか知りたいと思う
(l. 10) I wish S could have 過去分詞　S が～だったらよかったのに　　(l. 12) slide　悪化
(l. 12) no longer ~　もはや～でない　　(l. 13) acknowledge　認める　　(l. 15) widow　未亡人　　(l. 16) afterward　後で
(l. 17) stick　動かなくなる　　(l. 18) find oneself ~ing　自分が～しているのに気づく　　(l. 18) measure　判断する
(l. 18) questioner　質問者　　(l. 19) seem to ~　～するように思われる　　(l. 23) meanwhile　対照的に
(l. 23) on the rise　上昇中で　　(l. 27) have power over ~　～を支配する　　(l. 28) acquaintance　知り合い
(l. 28) late　最近亡くなった

Reading Comprehension

次の英文が，本文の内容と一致する場合は T，一致しない場合は F を選びなさい。

1. (T / F) Elena worked with pediatric AIDS patients in Florida.
2. (T / F) Clarence didn't want anyone to see Elena as an AIDS patient's wife.
3. (T / F) Ryan White was prohibited from going to school because he was an AIDS patient.
4. (T / F) Elena shared her own story with Jasmine's mother.
5. (T / F) After Clarence's death, Elena didn't have to keep secrets, so she shared her own story at the support group meeting.

EXERCISES　**Dictation & Translation**　　CD 2-29 ▶ 69

音声を聴いて英文の空欄に適語を記入しなさい。また，完成した英文を日本語に直しなさい。

1. He _____ _____ _____ prostate cancer last year.

   _____

2. She _____ _____ _____ discuss the details.

   _____

3. I _____ _____ he knows we're here.

   _____

4. The effect _____ _____ last about thirty minutes.

   _____

5. Inflation is _____ _____ _____ again.

   _____

EXERCISES　**Word Order & Translation**　　CD 2-30 ▶ 70

日本文の意味に合うように，（　）内の語句を並べかえて英文を作りなさい。

1. 外国人ジャーナリストはその国に入ることを禁止されていた。

   (were / the country / from / journalists / entering / barred / foreign).

   _____

2. 彼女は両親に連絡を取ろうと努力しなかった。

   (her parents / to / no / she / contact / effort / made).

   _____

3. そんなにたくさん食べなければよかった。

   (hadn't / I / so / wish / much / eaten / I).

   _____

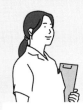

LEARN MORE

Nursing Terms and Expressions

次の日本文の空欄に入る語を下から選びなさい。

黄疸，　過食症，　合併症，　失禁，　湿疹，　褥瘡，　低体温症，　不眠症

じょくそう

1. Anorexia and **bulimia** are the most common eating disorders.
   拒食症と＿＿＿＿＿＿＿は，最もよくある摂食障害だ。

2. Once a **bedsore** develops, it is often very slow to heal.
   いったん＿＿＿＿＿＿＿ができると，治癒するのがたいていの場合とても遅い。

3. Sometimes, **complications** can occur after surgery.
   時々，手術後に＿＿＿＿＿＿＿が起こる場合がある。

4. Atopic dermatitis is the most common type of **eczema**.
   アトピー性皮膚炎は，最もよくあるタイプの＿＿＿＿＿＿＿だ。

5. A person with severe **hypothermia** may be unconscious.
   ひどい＿＿＿＿＿＿＿の人は，意識不明になるかもしれない。

6. There are several types of urinary **incontinence**.
   尿＿＿＿＿＿＿＿には，いくつかのタイプがある。

7. My father suffered from **insomnia** caused by stress at work.
   私の父は，職場のストレスが原因の＿＿＿＿＿＿＿に苦しんでいた。

8. Babies with **jaundice** have a yellow coloring of the skin and eyes.
   ＿＿＿＿＿＿＿にかかった赤ちゃんは，皮膚と目の色が黄色い。

Column

　vital signs の sign は，Babinski sign（バビンスキー徴候）や Wernicke sign（ウェルニッケ徴候）のように，医学用語では「徴候」という意味で使われることが多い語です。この sign を使った興味深いスラング表現があります。

　O sign と Q sign は，いずれも患者の状態を視覚的にとらえた表現です。患者の口が O の文字のようにポカンと空いている様子が O sign，その口から舌がだらりと出ている状態が Q sign です。いずれも患者の容体が芳しくない場合に使われる表現です。

　positive suitcase sign は，入院の必要のない患者が，身の回り品を入れたスーツケースを持ち，入院を期待して繰り返し病院に姿を現す状況を指しています。「陽性の」という意味の positive を付けていかにも医学用語のような響きにしています。週末に出かける家族から見放された高齢者が行き場を失ってやってくる場合もあり，高齢者社会の悲しい現実を表す表現でもあります。

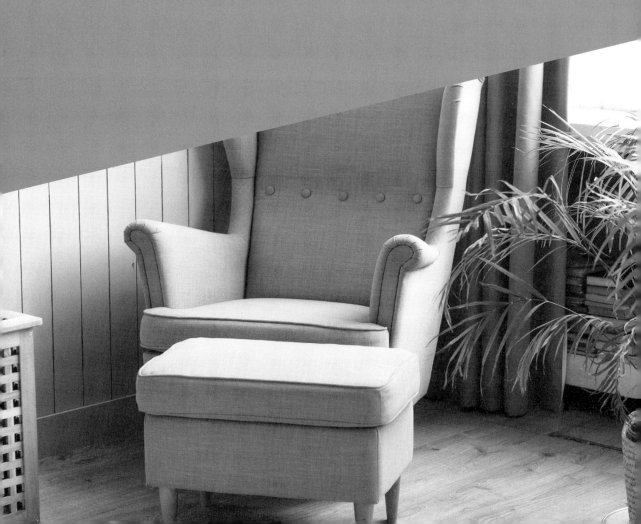

Unit 15

A Man of Few Words

What we don't know about our patients.

Kathryn Mason, MSN, RN, PCCN

次の英語の意味に合う日本語を下から選びなさい。また，音声を聴いて発音しなさい。

1. deficit　　_____

2. wound　　_____

3. countenance　_____

4. hesitation　_____

5. utterance　_____

創傷，発言，表情，躊躇，障害

READING　**Essay【Part 1】**　CD 2-32 ▶ 72

エッセイの出だしを読んでみましょう。

Medical and Nursing Notes

Willy had a long last name that we believed to be of Hungarian or Czechoslovakian descent; however, this was purely conjecture. We really didn't know his country of origin, and Willy wasn't talking.

5　Willy had suffered a debilitating stroke some years earlier and his most striking deficit was profound expressive aphasia. He was unable to articulate more than a few errant words at a time and most of the time his speech consisted of garbled, unintelligible sounds. Willy's affliction belied an otherwise

10　sturdy appearance for a man in his late 70s. He had carved features, with a strong, square chin and gnarled hands that hinted of an earlier life filled with manual labor. I privately imagined that, before his stroke, he had spoken with an accent and a cadence similar to those of Arnold Schwarzenegger.

suffer　（苦痛などを）経験する
stroke　脳卒中
profound　重度の
expressive　表出性の
aphasia　失語症
articulate　はっきり発音する

chin　あご

Notes　(l. 2) descent　家系　　(l. 3) conjecture　推測　　(l. 5) debilitating　衰弱させるような
(l. 7) be unable to ~　~することができない　　(l. 7) errant　誤った　　(l. 7) at a time　一度に，同時に
(l. 8) most of the time　ほとんどの場合は　　(l. 8) consist of ~　~から成る　　(l. 8) garbled　意味不明の
(l. 9) unintelligible　理解できない　　(l. 9) affliction　苦悩　　(l. 9) belie　誤った印象を与える
(l. 9) otherwise　違ったふうに　　(l. 10) sturdy　たくましい　　(l. 10) carved　彫刻されたような
(l. 11) square　角張った　　(l. 11) gnarled　こぶだらけの　　(l. 12) hint of ~　~を暗示する
(l. 12) manual labor　肉体労働　　(l. 13) accent　なまり　　(l. 14) cadence　抑揚

Check the situation

Q1 ウィリーのラストネームから推測されることは？

Q2 ウィリーは病気になる前にどのような仕事をしていたと考えられるか？

Our home care agency had maintained Willy on service for several months, treating a nonhealing diabetic wound on his foot. The home health nurses were his only resource: we filled his medication box and made certain that there was
5　food in the house through the Meals on Wheels program (or by bringing food on our visits). The agency provided a home health aide and generally looked after his safety and well-being. It was an unspoken understanding that Willy wouldn't be discharged from services in the near future. We were all willing
10　accomplices.

For a time, I was assigned to be the primary RN on the case. The nursing care plan called for dressing changes to the foot four to five times per week. I made at least three of those visits each week and my routine with Willy became fairly rote.
15　He sat in the same chair each time, with his foot propped on an ottoman; I was positioned in front of the foot, my back to his decrepit television. I would chatter away to compensate for his lack of dialogue, regaling him with stories of my children, the weather, or whatever other bits of news came to mind.
20　Sometimes he would give me his rapt attention and at other times he would be more intent on the news or a game show.

On Labor Day weekend 1997, I found myself unexpectedly having to cover patient visits. It was to have been a day off for me and I was annoyed at this sudden change in plans. My
25　family was enjoying a barbecue and company at home while I was traversing rural roads, visiting homebound patients. Like Willy.

Medical and Nursing Notes

home care　在宅ケア

nonhealing　治らない
diabetic　糖尿病性の
home health nurse　訪問看護師

medication box　薬収納ケース

Meals on Wheels　ミールズ・オン・ホイールズ（老人や病人に対する食事の宅配サービス）
home health aide　ホームヘルパー

primary　プライマリー（一人の患者を入院から退院までの全期間を通して継続的に受け持つ）
RN　登録看護師（registered nurse）
dressing change　包帯交換（dressing は創傷被覆材のこと）

Notes　(l. 3) resource　（いざという時の）頼み　　(l. 4) make certain that ~　～であることを確かめる
(l. 7) look after ~　～に気をつける　　(l. 9) discharge　解放する　　(l. 9) in the near future　そのうち
(l. 9) willing accomplice　自発的な共犯者　　(l. 11) for a time　しばらくの間　　(l. 12) call for ~　～を必要とする
(l. 13) at least　少なくとも　　(l. 14) rote　機械的な反復　　(l. 15) prop　支える
(l. 16) ottoman　（クッションつき）足台　　(l. 16) in front of ~　～の前に　　(l. 17) decrepit　おんぼろの
(l. 17) chatter away　しゃべり続ける　　(l. 17) compensate for ~　～の埋め合わせをする　　(l. 18) regale　楽しませる
(l. 19) bits of ~　わずかな～　　(l. 19) come to mind　思い浮かぶ
(l. 20) sometimes ~ at other times ...　ある時には～またある時には…　　(l. 20) rapt　うっとりした
(l. 21) be intent on ~　～に没頭している　　(l. 21) game show　ゲーム番組
(l. 22) Labor Day　（米国・カナダ）労働者の日　　(l. 22) find oneself ~ing　自分が～しているのに気づく
(l. 22) unexpectedly　思いがけなく　　(l. 24) be annoyed at ~　～にむっとしている
(l. 25) company　一緒にいること　　(l. 26) homebound　外出できない

Willy was my last visit of the day. When I arrived, he was already ensconced in his chair, awaiting my arrival. He didn't seem to notice my stormy countenance or my marked silence. While I worked on his foot, he continued to watch the news in
5　silence (which somehow irritated me even more). As I neared the end of my task, Willy's foot inexplicably became a squirmy moving target that I was struggling to dress in gauze wrap. Head bent over the foot, determined to swiftly complete the task and head home, I found my attention suddenly arrested by
10　a rich male voice: "The Lady died."

　　I whipped around to see who had entered the home undetected, but no one was there. Suddenly, I knew—Willy. He had spoken those three words to me, without impediment or hesitation. As I looked incredulously into his face, I realized that
15　he was pointing at the television behind me, where the tragic news of the death of the Princess of Wales had broken into the regularly scheduled program.

　　On shaking legs, I sank to the ottoman. To this day, I don't know if I was more stunned by the news of Princess Diana or by
20　Willy's unexpected utterance. He was clearly shaken and moved by the death, and I found myself deeply ashamed of my earlier display of petulance. I moved a chair next to his and took his hand. We watched the news of the accident in Paris for about an hour in silence. Willy spoke no more that day, nor did I ever
25　again hear him clearly speak understandable language.

　　Driving home later that afternoon, it occurred to me that Willy had spoken without a trace of accent, Hungarian or otherwise.

dress　包帯をする
gauze wrap　ガーゼラップ

impediment　言語障害

Notes　(l. 1) be ensconced　座っている　　(l. 3) stormy　激しい　　(l. 3) marked　著しい　　(l. 4) work on ~　~に取り組む
(l. 4) in silence　黙って　　(l. 5) somehow　どういうわけか　　(l. 5) irritate　いらいらさせる
(l. 6) inexplicably　どういうわけか　　(l. 6) squirmy　身もだえする　　(l. 7) moving target　動く標的
(l. 7) struggle to ~　~しようと苦労する　　(l. 8) bend over　身をかがめる　　(l. 8) determined　固く決心した
(l. 8) swiftly　速やかに　　(l. 9) arrest　引く　　(l. 11) whip around　急に振り向く
(l. 12) undetected　気づかれていない　　(l. 14) incredulously　疑い深く　　(l. 15) point at ~　~を指さす
(l. 16) Princess of Wales　(the ~)　ザ・プリンセス・オブ・ウエールズ（英国皇太子妃の称号）
(l. 18) to this day　今日まで　　(l. 19) stunned　愕然として　　(l. 22) petulance　不機嫌　　(l. 22) next to ~　~の隣に
(l. 26) it occurs to A that ~　A の心に~が浮かぶ　　(l. 27) a trace of ~　~ほんの少しの ~
(l. 27) or otherwise　あるいは他の

Reading Comprehension

次の英文が，本文の内容と一致する場合は T，一致しない場合は F を選びなさい。

1. (T / F) The home care agency didn't have to provide home care to Willy.
2. (T / F) Willy needed dressing changes to the foot three times a week.
3. (T / F) When Kathryn (the writer) visited Willy, she was irritated because she couldn't enjoy a barbecue with her family.
4. (T / F) At first, Kathryn didn't know who spoke the three words.
5. (T / F) Willy and Kathryn talked about the news of Princess Dianna for about an hour.

EXERCISES **Dictation & Translation** CD 2-34 ▶ 74

音声を聴いて英文の空欄に適語を記入しなさい。また，完成した英文を日本語に直しなさい。

1. I can only do one thing _____ _____ _____.

   _____

2. Who's going to _____ _____ the children tomorrow?

   _____

3. He _____ _____ _____ himself for making such a mistake.

   _____

4. I need to _____ _____ my essay.

   _____

5. There was _____ _____ _____ poison in the cup.

   _____

EXERCISES **Word Order & Translation** CD 2-35 ▶ 75

日本文の意味に合うように，（ ）内の語句を並べかえて英文を作りなさい。

1. その委員会は，医師，看護師，ソーシャルワーカーで構成されている。

   (social workers / nurses / of / the committee / and / doctors / consists).

   _____

2. あなたはすべて整っていることを確かめるべきだ。

   (order / everything / make / in / that / should / certain / you / is).

   _____

3. 自分の妻が幸せでないかもしれないという考えは，トムの心には浮かばなかった。

   (occurred / unhappy / his wife / to / it / might / Tom / never / be / that).

   _____

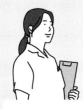

Nursing Terms and Expressions

次の英文の空欄に入る語を下から選びなさい。

> constipation, delirium, hangover, hypertension, indigestion, palpitations, pneumonia, sore throat

1. My grandmother nearly died of _____.
私の祖母は，**肺炎**で死ぬところだった。

2. If I eat onions, they give me _____.
タマネギを食べると，私は**消化不良**を起こす。

3. She woke up with a bad _____.
彼女は，ひどい**二日酔い**で目覚めた。

4. She coughed a lot, so she has a _____.
咳がたくさん出るので，彼女は**のどが痛い**。

5. The patient was very sick and in a _____.
その患者は，とても具合が悪くて**譫妄状態**だった。

6. Caffeine can cause headaches and heart _____.
カフェインが原因で，頭痛や心臓の**動悸**が起こることがある。

7. He takes medicine to lower _____.
高血圧を下げるために，彼は薬を服用している。

8. Iron supplements may cause stomach problems, such as heartburn, nausea, diarrhea, and _____.
鉄分サプリメントは，胸やけ，吐き気，下痢，**便秘**のような胃の問題を起こすかもしれない。

Column

　言葉の滑稽な誤用のことをマラプロピズム（malapropism）と呼びます。18 世紀の戯曲『恋がたき』（The Rivals）の中でよく言い間違えをする登場人物 Mrs. Malaprop の名前に由来します。このように，ある言葉を他の似ている言葉と間違えてしまうことは医学用語の場合にも起こり，例えば，palpitation を population（人口），pneumonia を ammonia（アンモニア），fibroid（子宮筋腫）を fireball（火の玉），Alzheimer's disease（アルツハイマー病）を old timer's disease（古参病）と言ったりします。では，次の語と間違えられた語を下から選び，その意味を調べてみましょう。

1. inflation（インフレーション）　　2. legend（伝説）　　3. service（サービス）

4. very close veins（非常に近い静脈）　5. vowel movement（母音の動き）

> bowel movement, cervix, inflammation, lesion, varicose veins

編著者
田中芳文（たなか　よしふみ）　島根県立大学人間文化学部教授

看護師たちのリフレクション
—医療現場のストーリーで学ぶ英語—

─────────────────────────────

2023 年 2 月 20 日　第 1 版発行

編　著　者──田中芳文
発　行　者──前田俊秀
発　行　所──株式会社　三修社
　　　　　　　〒 150-0001　東京都渋谷区神宮前 2-2-22
　　　　　　　TEL 03-3405-4511 / FAX 03-3405-4522
　　　　　　　振替 00190-9-72758
　　　　　　　https://www.sanshusha.co.jp
　　　　　　　編集担当　三井るり子・伊藤宏実

印　刷　所──港北メディアサービス株式会社

─────────────────────────────

©2023 Printed in Japan　ISBN978-4-384-33519-4　C1082

表紙デザイン —NONdesign
Ｄ　Ｔ　Ｐ —Office haru
準拠音声制作 —高速録音株式会社
準拠音声録音 —ELEC（吹込：Josh Keller / Jennifer Okano）